Reviews—Healing Through Empathy

I was personally touched by the kindness, empathy, and expertise that Dr Adams showed the patients in his book. It should be mandatory that every medical student read *Healing Through Empathy*.
James Avery, MD
Medical Director
VNSNY Hospice Care

Healing Through Empathy is a great read and an inspiring book. As a physical therapist working with physically challenged children, I found Dr. Adams' book enlightening and have recommended it to my colleagues as well as to the parents of my patients.
Lisa Haid, RPT

Anyone facing a major health issue or those in the profession looking for a better approach will find *Healing Through Empathy* an invaluable addition to their library.
Shirley Roe
Allbooks Reviews

Healing Through Empathy

Healing Through Empathy

Francis V. Adams, M.D.

iUniverse, Inc.
New York Lincoln Shanghai

Healing Through Empathy

iUniverse books may be ordered through booksellers or by contacting:

iUniverse
2021 Pine Lake Road, Suite 100
Lincoln, NE 68512
www.iuniverse.com
1-800-Authors (1-800-288-4677)

ISBN: 0-595-31626-3 (pbk)
ISBN: 0-595-66345-1 (cloth)

Printed in the United States of America

In memory of my friend and colleague, Peter Pasternack, M.D., who cared for so many and for my wife, Laura Anne, who has given new meaning to my life.

Contents

INTRODUCTION

In many ways, our health care system is in turmoil. Surveys of patients and physicians reveal widespread dissatisfaction. Patients are dissatisfied with the failure of their physicians to communicate. In addition, they face an increasingly complex and expensive health care industry. Physicians are dissatisfied with managed care and the lack of time they have to spend with individual patients. The end result of this mutual dissatisfaction is often a bad outcome to a patient's illness.

The purpose of this book is to illustrate through actual case histories the importance of communication between physicians and patients and to demonstrate how this vital relationship affects the diagnosis, treatment and outcome of an illness. Although communication between physicians and patients has been stressed before, this book allows the reader to "step into" consultation and examination rooms to observe firsthand the interaction of a doctor and his patients. From witnessing the medical experiences of others, the reader will be better equipped to choose who their physician should be. The Appendix includes further information on how to choose a physician and find out more about specific illnesses discussed in this book.

In the practice of medicine, physicians learn that there is a wonderful, natural balance of the human body and its chemistry of health and life. Medicine advances daily to further prolong life and achieve miracles but a doctor quickly recognizes that death is natural and inevitable. The science of medicine has advanced rapidly to a better understanding of the functioning of the human body. At the same time, the art of healing and the role of the primary physician have been diminished. This book describes seven patients in whom the doctor-patient relationship played a major role in diagnosis, treatment, and outcome. In many of the cases I describe, a patient and medicine triumph over illness, but in others death is the victor. In all of the cases, the human spirit and the role of empathy in healing are revealed.

Doctors have been known as "healers" long before the introduction of medicines and surgery and certainly prior to achieving many successful cures. The art of healing requires vital communication between physician and patient. This exchange is of sensations and knowledge that may lead to empathy and understanding and forms the basis of diagnosis and treatment. Communication may occur through all of our senses including touch but requires an investment of time that in the current managed care era is sorely lacking. The rushed physician of the 21st century tends to rely more on technology to tell him what is wrong with his patient rather than what he may learn through his senses.

Medical students and young physicians have long been told to "not get involved emotionally" with their patients since that would destroy their objectivity. This often produces physicians who appear cold and detached without a trace of empathy. Faced with illness and suffering it is impossible not to be moved, especially as a physician seeking to provide care and relief. Empathy is much more than sympathy for another person's pain and suffering. It is the ability to visualize mental images and to instantly recognize moods so that one individual can sense the emotions of another. Above all, empathy requires interest and communication. In a long association between doctor and patient life experiences are shared and a bond may strengthen through the diagnosis and treatment of a serious illness. A patient I have treated for 20 years said to me recently, "You're my doctor but I feel that you are also my friend."

I often tell patients and their families that you get to know an individual very quickly as a physician treating a serious illness. A person's character is severely tested by a dire diagnosis, endless and exhausting tests, institutionalized loss of dignity, pain, and anxiety. By listening to my patients' histories and seeing how they react to such circumstances, I have found that I've gained a greater understanding of my patients and of myself. The empathy that I have realized with my patients has provided me with further insight into their state of mind. This open communication provides knowledge useful in diagnosis and promotes the development of the best treatment plan. In this way, empathy may empower a physician to achieve the best outcome, to truly "heal," if not cure.

I began my medical career at Cornell Medical College in 1967 but my medical education started long before that. My father, Vincent J. Adams, was an Internist and Cardiologist who practiced medicine for more than forty years. He met my mother, Rose, a nurse, during his internship and fell in love instantly. They married, and despite a six-year stint in the armed services (1940–1946), including a D-Day landing, they managed to start a family of three children. The atmosphere in our home was charged with medicine. Some of my earliest memories are of my dad, on the phone with his patients and other physicians, often answering emergency calls in the middle of dinner or leaving at all hours for the hospital or a patient's home. After church on Sundays he would often take the three of us to the hospital where we would wait until he finished rounds. I have no doubt that this environment created my desire to become a physician. I wasn't the only one affected. My sister, Julie, is a clinical psychologist who practices in Lexington, VA. and my brother, Peter, is a cardiothoracic surgeon.

After graduation from Cornell in 1971, I became an intern at Georgetown University Hospital in Washington, D.C. and completed my medical residency there in 1973. I then entered a two-year fellowship program in pulmonary disease at Bellevue Hospital Center in New York City. In 1977, board-certified in Internal Medicine and Pulmonary Disease, I entered private practice. Medicine has given me the opportunity to attempt to extend life and in many instances, succeed. There is no greater experience than to see an individual restored to good health.

This book also reveals many of the emotions experienced by a doctor. I remember witnessing, as a medical student, the last few minutes of a patient's life. I had seen corpses and had participated in the dissection of a cadaver but had never actually seen someone die. Death can be silent, like falling off to sleep but my first experience was an agonizing death of a cancer patient. I was shaken and left with the strong impression that my role must also be to decrease and prevent suffering.

The current outcry from patients that physicians are cold, unfeeling, and that they do not listen, must be heard. Changes in medical school curriculums that require medical students to take on the role of patients and begin their bedside training earlier are important steps toward "humanizing" doctors. Increased recognition by insurance companies of the value of office and hospital visits as opposed to procedures is essential for a proper balance of the art and science of medicine to be restored.

The seven cases I have recorded here are offered to provide insight into the doctor-patient relationship. Patient names and small details have been changed in order to ensure privacy. Although these case histories are unusual and may provide interesting material, they are not unique. Every physician has seen extraordinary and challenging patients and made difficult diagnoses. It is my hope that these pages will reveal that in dealing with patients physicians do not have to be detached and may achieve more by recognizing rather than suppressing their emotional response.

I am indebted to two special individuals without whom this book would not have been written. Mary Kane, my patient but also a dear friend, provided tremendous support for this project. My extraordinary wife, Laura Anne, inspired me to finish this book and to make it better. Above all I am indebted to my patients who have given me their trust and the privilege of caring for them.

1

Sleep, Sweet Sleep

I have been the fortunate student of great diagnosticians, always hoping to learn techniques from them that would assist me with my own patients. One of these doctors was my father, Dr. Vincent J. Adams, who took me on house calls and hospital rounds when I was in my teens.

My dad loved people and conversation. After first engaging his patients in discussion, he then proceeded quickly and deftly to examine them. At the end of a conversation he could often tell the patient what the problem was. Though he had large hands, his was an extremely light touch. A common patient response was, "But you haven't examined me yet!"

My conclusions were that my father and other talented physicians that I studied under had three gifts in common: Extremely sharp senses, empathy for their fellow man, and intuition. Although technology has reached incredible levels, diagnostic ability is still greatly intuitive. Like Big Blue programmed to play chess against the grand masters, computer hard drives are now filled with medical information and programmed to make diagnoses, but they lack the three key characteristics I have noted. I doubt that machines will ever replace an intuitive doctor at the bedside.

Louis Goodman touched all of my senses when I first encountered him. It was by sound rather than sight that I found him, and it wouldn't have been necessary to have had good hearing!

The year was 1974. I was in the second year of my pulmonary fellow-ship and my assignment was consulting at the Manhattan Veterans Administration Hospital. I would receive requests for consultation from various services throughout the hospital, see the patient in question, and then discuss the case with an attending physician. This particular day I was to see Mr. Goodman on the 12th floor of the hospital.

As I approached the 12th floor nursing station where the patient charts are kept, I became aware of a very loud noise. In Manhattan, construction and street repair are daily events so at first I thought the commotion must have been coming from outside the hospital. Was it perhaps a buzz saw? Just as I was about to investigate further, the noise stopped abruptly, so I went on to enter the nursing station and located the chart labeled, "GOODMAN, Louis."

As I opened the chart I heard a loud grunting sound followed by the same excruciatingly loud noise. I knew I had come closer to the source since the sound was more intense and concluded it was coming from within the hospital. Although I might have imagined it, to this day I believe the reverberations of this annoying sound sent off vibrations that were bouncing off the walls. Then it stopped again.

As one of the nurses passed by, I stopped her to ask, "What's that terrible noise?"

"Oh that's Goodman. He snores. Some of us are using earplugs. They say his wife brought him here because she couldn't stand it anymore. He's in room 1204 down the hall."

I didn't have to check the room numbers to locate him. The noise led me. Just as I entered his room, it stopped again. Room 1204 was a small single hospital room, measuring about 12x10 feet. I literally squeezed myself inside the door for Mr. Goodman seemed to fill the room entirely. He was huge. I estimated upwards of 350 pounds were piled upon a height of about 5 feet, 6 inches. His color was blue. Very blue, a sign of a low blood oxygen level or cyanosis. The patient appeared to be asleep but as I approached him I realized he was not breathing. The medical term for the cessation of breathing is *apnea*.

Just as I pondered an appropriate action, his whole body shuddered and he let out a loud grunt, opened his eyes and demanded crossly, "Who are you?" I noticed that his color began to improve immediately, and while observing him closely, I introduced myself.

I asked, "Do you know that you snore?"

"That's what they say, but I think they're making it up. My wife complains and complains but I think she just wants to sleep in another room. She said to me, 'If you don't go to the hospital and get something done about that snoring, I'm leaving you.' If she weren't such a good cook, I would have let her leave. So here I am." I could tell by looking at him that she must indeed be a very good cook.

As he finished the sentence, his eyes closed, and within a moment he was asleep and snoring again. I watched him for the next few minutes and saw his color again become blue and his breathing and snoring come to a halt. I tapped him several times on the shoulder.

He awoke with a start, saying, "You're still here? Can you get me something to eat? The food in this hospital is terrible."

I tried humor. "My assignment is to assist the other doctors with your case, not supervise the kitchen, however bad the food. Maybe we could have your wife give the chef some tips."

I attempted to take his medical history, but it was slow going since Mr. Goodman would listen to my questions, answer partially and immediately fall back asleep. I tapped him awake again and again.

"Do you know that you have trouble staying awake?"

"Yeah, I seem to nod off a lot. Once I fell asleep at the wheel of my car." I had trouble picturing him squeeze his 350 pounds into an automobile when he added, "That was when I was only 250 pounds and able to drive. Lately, I can't seem to get out of the house".

After about an hour I was able to piece together Mr. Goodman's history. He was 54 years old, and he had seen action in Europe during WW II. After the war he started his own business but had been unable to work for the last year and a half. Then I found some common ground. He loved baseball, as did I, and we found that we both rooted for the Mets.

"I watch the games but I seem to fall asleep before they end," he complained. Louis also admitted he had always had a weight problem that had worsened in the last few years, gaining nearly 60 pounds. I learned that he had had high blood pressure for a few years, and he was taking medication prescribed by his internist. For the last two to three years his family had observed that he would often fall asleep during the day and the incident while driving his car had occurred about two years earlier.

I also spoke to his wife, who had somehow managed to squeeze into the room with us. She reported that he had always snored but it had become so bad in the last few years so that she now slept in a separate bedroom.

"It doesn't make much difference. You can still hear him in any part of the house. We can't have houseguests. No one will stay over because I swear the walls shake. Please do something," she pleaded.

Mrs. Goodman described the same pattern that I had observed. There were periods during the nights when her husband appeared not to be breathing followed by grunting noises and "shaking."

After obtaining the medical history, I gave him a physical examination that revealed Mr. Goodman's blood pressure was elevated (160/100; normal is 110/70) and that his pulse was irregular. I also noted that his breath sounds were diminished in intensity, his heart appeared to be enlarged and his legs were swollen.

My next steps were to review his chest x-rays, EKG, and laboratory tests. I would need all of this information to present to the attending physician with whom I would discuss this absorbing case. The Goodmans had now engaged both my professional expertise and my concern. I wanted to be able to help.

My patient's x-ray and EKG did indeed reveal an enlarged heart, which I concluded might be due to his high blood pressure. Blood gas analysis confirmed that while he was sleeping Mr. Goodman's blood oxygen level was only 48 (normal 80–100) and when awake it increased to 58. His blood work showed an elevated red blood cell count that I attributed to the lowered blood oxygen level. Red blood cells contain the oxygen-carrying protein known as *hemoglobin*. As oxygen levels drop, production of a hormone known as *erythropoetin* increases, stimulating the blood marrow to produce more new red blood cells. This compensatory increase in red cells increases the amount of oxygen reaching the body's organs.

My conclusion was that Louis Goodman suffered from a condition known as sleep apnea. This sleep disorder has been known for more than 100 years but most of the information about sleep apnea has been obtained in the last 30 years. It is estimated to occur in about 5 percent of adult men but is uncommon in pre-menopausal women. The frequency of sleep apnea in post-menopausal women, however, nearly equals that of adult men. Apnea is defined as an absence of air movement at the nose or mouth for at least ten seconds. This phenomenon is not always abnormal since sleep studies have documented that adults may have as many as five apneas per hour.

In patients with the sleep apnea syndrome, apneas occur much more frequently and for longer time periods. In severe cases, such as that of Louis Goodman, the apneas may last for sixty to ninety seconds and may recur up to five hundred times a night.

More than 90 percent of sleep apneas occur due to a closure of the muscles that support the throat. These muscles normally maintain the throat's air passage opening so that their closure effectively shuts or obstructs the breathing passageway. This form of sleep apnea is called *obstructive*. The remaining 10 percent of sleep apnea occurs when the respiratory center in the brain fails to trigger breathing and is referred to as *central*. Most individuals with obstructive sleep apnea (OSA) are overweight and many are obese. Obesity is defined by body weight that is 20 percent over the ideal predicted by age and sex. Although the relationship between obesity and sleep apnea is not clearly defined, the frequency of sleep-disordered breathing increases with weight gain. In many patients with the syndrome, improvement results from weight reduction.

Normal sleep occurs in stages of decreased consciousness. In general, sleep can be divided into "quiet" or non-rapid eye movement sleep (non-REM) and "active" rapid eye movement sleep (REM). In adults, REM sleep accounts for 25 percent of sleep time. Most dreams occur during REM sleep, which also may exhibit twitching movements of the face and limbs. During sleep, breathing becomes shallower. As a result of smaller breaths, oxygen levels decrease and carbon dioxide levels rise. Sensors located in the brain and neck regulate breathing and continue to respond to these changes but do so more slowly, particularly during REM sleep.

In the normal individual, the smaller breaths and changes in blood gas levels during sleep have little physical effect. Alcohol, tranquilizers, and sleeping pills, however, may exaggerate these changes and severely depress breathing. In patients with breathing disorders, the change in breathing patterns during sleep is more pronounced producing increased symptoms, as when oxygen levels fall to very low levels.

Sleep deprivation has been shown to be detrimental to human beings. Sleep, particularly REM sleep, appears to be essential for normal body function. Patients with obstructive sleep apnea (OSA) are sleep-deprived due to a pattern of repeated apneas followed by awakening.

As demonstrated so vividly by Mr. Goodman, the stoppage of breathing produces a drop in oxygen level and a rise in carbon dioxide. These changes cause alarm signals to be sent to centers in the brain which respond by producing arousal. The patient then falls asleep again and repeats the same cycle over and over during the night. This severely fragmented sleep pattern produces the excessive sleepiness or somnolence during the day.

The tendency to fall asleep during the day is the most common symptom of sleep apnea. One of the consequences of daytime hypersomnolence is a greater frequency of automobile accidents. Decreased productivity at work has also been documented. A number of other medical problems are now also directly connected to sleep apnea. These include high blood pressure, strokes, and heart attacks. The pressure within the blood vessels of the lung may also rise producing a strain on the heart muscle that may lead to heart failure. A common manifestation of this, as illustrated by Louis Goodman, is fluid retention producing swelling of the legs.

Loud snoring is the second most common symptom of OSA. Snoring results from narrowing of the air passageway of the nose and throat. It is more common in adults and increases with age. Snoring may occur without sleep apnea.

In order to diagnose sleep apnea, a formal sleep study is required and I arranged for Mr. Goodman to be studied the next night. Sleep studies, called polysomnography, are performed overnight with monitoring of brain activity, the flow of air at the patient's mouth, chest movements, EKG, and oxygen levels. I explained the study to my patient and told him that he would wear a number of monitoring devices.

"I'll never be able to sleep," he said. "You can forget about it."

When I asked him if he ever dreamed he answered a little wistfully, I thought.

"You know, it's been years. When I was a kid, I loved to play ball and in my dreams I made the big leagues. It's funny. I sleep but I don't dream much."

I told him we would be recording his brain waves during the sleep study and that many people with his condition don't dream because they never reach a certain level of sleep.

"Let me know what you find, Doc, but I still don't think I'll be able to sleep with those wires on my head."

In 1974 the VA Hospital did not yet have a formal sleep laboratory. Instead, the brain monitoring equipment was brought to the patient's bedside and I participated in setting up the monitors. With all of the equipment, my patient, a technician, and two other physicians, there was literally no room to turn around in room 1204. For a second I wondered myself if anyone could sleep under these conditions.

I was wrong. Mr. Goodman fell asleep before the last electrode was attached to his scalp and his snoring began. Forewarned, we had all come with earplugs but the noise still seemed to reverberate off the four walls of his room. We began to collect the data, each of us responsible for monitoring one piece of equipment.

I graphed the airflow at Louis's mouth as well as the movement of his chest muscles and quickly saw the characteristic pattern of OSA. My patient's apneas were clearly of the obstructive type since I could see that the flow of air at his mouth stopped while his chest wall muscles continued to move. This meant that the brain centers were still firing signals for him to breathe and that the apnea must be due to the closure of his throat muscles.

In some patients the blockage in the throat is due to another type of abnormality such as very large tonsils or a congenital deformity. The flap of tissue that hangs down the back of the throat is called the *uvula*. In some individuals with OSA, a recently developed treatment includes trimming away excessive tissue in the back of the throat and shortening the uvula. This surgical procedure may improve the condition in 50 percent of patients with OSA. All patients with sleep apnea also undergo a careful examination of his or her upper airway, looking for an abnormality that can be corrected surgically.

My patient's sleep study lasted for three hours. During this time period, Mr. Goodman had several hundred apneas and his oxygen levels dropped repeatedly to the 40s. The brain wave study revealed that he never reached REM sleep and that he was repeatedly aroused by the changes in his blood gases. At the end of the study, I tapped him on the shoulder to wake him.

As he woke, he crowed, "I told you I would never sleep with all these wires and people in my room. I guess you'll have to find another way." I finally convinced him that he had truly slept through the test.

I discussed the findings and treatment plan with the attending physician. Although a number of effective treatments are currently prescribed for sleep apnea, in 1974, the treatment options were extremely limited. One option was to prescribe medications that would stimulate the breathing center, for instance progesterone, a female hormone. The use of this medication had grown out of observations of women during pregnancy who exhibited increased rates of breathing. Its use in OSA proved only mildly effective, however. Other medications such as nervous system stimulants were also tried but provided minimal benefits. Weight reduction was encouraged but proved very difficult to achieve by most patients.

Today OSA is treated with an air pressure device called CPAP that uses the flow of air to maintain the opening of the throat, but in 1974 the most effective treatment was a tracheotomy. This is a minor surgical procedure in which an opening is created in the windpipe below the level of the throat and a tube inserted to maintain the opening. The tube effectively bypasses the obstruction to the upper airway that occurs when the muscles of the throat close.

A tracheotomy is not without drawbacks, which I explained to Louis Goodman. One of the most distressing is interference with normal speech since it is the rush of air past the vocal cords that creates voice. The tracheotomy tube would eliminate speaking normally. In addition, swallowing difficulties may occur after a tracheotomy and there is also the risk of infection as well as the need to suction out a buildup of mucus in the tube.

I explained these adverse effects to Mr. Goodman and stressed that he would be able to speak by plugging the tracheotomy tube, which would allow air to pass around it to vibrate the vocal cords. He could keep the tracheotomy tube plugged during the day and remove the plug at night when he was most at risk for apneas.

"I don't want a hole in my neck," he said. "It's not for me."

The harder I tried to convince him, the more adamant he became. I also spoke to his wife who was unable to convince him. "He can be pretty stubborn," she said.

Though I understood Louis's feelings, I was still convinced that the tracheotomy would improve his life immeasurably. How could I make him see it without proof? I didn't know that serendipity would step in.

The next day I was assigned to the Chest Clinic at the VA Hospital where I saw outpatients with pulmonary problems. Many of these men I was seeing for the first time. When I arrived I found a stack of charts in my examination room; picking up the first chart, I stepped into waiting area and called out, "Mr. Lynch." I heard a chair fall over,-looked in the direction of the noise and saw two veterans trying to help a very obese man stand up. They righted him and he turned towards me. I was struck by his girth but it was what he did next that really got my attention.

He brought his right hand up to his neck and the end of a metal tracheotomy tube, covered its opening with his index finger, and said, 'That's me, Doc. Tom Lynch."

Mr. Thomas Lynch's history was very similar to my patient's and he had had a tracheotomy performed for OSA two months prior to this visit. I asked him how he was doing.

Covering the opening of his tracheotomy tube he said, "It took some getting used to and I really don't like it but I am no longer falling asleep during the day and all the swelling in my legs is gone. My family says they can finally get some sleep. They said the whole house used to rattle from my snoring."

I thought for a moment and then asked, "Would you mind coming up to the 12th floor and talking to one of my patients? He really needs the same procedure you had but he has refused it."

"I'll do it, Doc, but I can't promise anything."

We went up to room 1204 and I introduced the two veterans. "I'll leave the two of you alone and come back after I finish my clinic rounds."

When I returned I found Mr. Lynch near the floor elevators.

"He's asleep now but I think he'll do it. My god, does he snore. He had a lot of questions and it turned out we were almost in the same outfit over-seas." He turned to enter one of the elevators but paused and said, "You know what I think convinced him? I told him that I was dreaming a lot more."

I thanked him and went down the hall to see my patient. He appeared to have just awakened as I entered.

"You don't give up, do you? Well, you can tell your surgeon friend to sharpen up his knife. I'll do it."

"You're doing the right thing. I'll have him come by to see you in the morning."

An Ear, Nose, and Throat surgeon performed a tracheotomy on Louis Goodman a few days later. After another week, with the tracheotomy tube in place, the sleep study was repeated. There was a marked improvement: Louis's oxygen level never fell below 55 and the number of apneas was drastically reduced. I also observed something that had not occurred during the first study.

While sleeping, Mr. Goodman exhibited rapid eye movements. I looked over at the technician monitoring his brain wave (EEG) tracing and he whispered to me, "It's REM, he's dreaming."

I looked at Louis's face and saw an expression of contentment I had not seen before. He had just hit a fastball out of the park.

Though the medical treatment is different today, the way of persuading a reluctant patient to try a proven therapy hasn't changed. In this case, introducing him to another patient in the same boat won the day and a brighter life for Louis Goodman.

As for me, I was left with the feeling that maybe I had some of my father's diagnostic gifts. I hoped so.

2

Walking Together

○ ○
"through the valley of the shadow…"

—*Psalm 23*

It is not unusual for a young person to bring a parent or relative or even a good friend to a doctor's appointment. The first time I met lovely young Mary Kelly, her mother and fiancé accompanied her. They all appeared nervous, and that was not unusual either—an initial visit to a doctor is never easy for any patient!

Other than being extremely slender, Mary had the glow of youth and did not appear ill. Only 22 years old, she had come to see me because she had had a severe cough for several months; she had already seen two physicians including another lung specialist, but had no relief from the coughing.

The four of us sat down in my consultation room for the preliminary interview. As we did, Mary coughed deeply and apologized.

"I can't help it."

I reassured her, saying I was sure we would get to the bottom of the problem.

She blurted, "I'm getting married in three months, so you have to get rid of my cough before then."

Though I smiled at her innocent confidence that I could accomplish what two other competent physicians had not been able to do, I was concerned. Time constraints on the speed of healing are not helpful either to the doctor or the patient. At that moment, I never considered the possibility that she would not survive until the wedding.

Age is one of the important factors that a physician considers when first interviewing a patient. Illnesses typically occur at different stages of life; this is especially true of certain forms of cancer. Just by knowing the patient's age and sex, the physician is able to narrow the possibilities that must be considered in any illness. Most patients in their early twenties who see a lung specialist are being treated for asthma or infections such as pneumonia.

Mary had been in good health all of her life, she said, and her mother confirmed that this was true. She had never smoked and had no allergies. About eight months prior to this visit the cough began. After a week of suffering from the problem, she visited her primary physician, who thought it was probably due to a cold or a post-nasal drip. Cough suppressant syrup and decongestant tablets were prescribed.

Mary returned to her physician two weeks later with the cough unrelieved. An x-ray was then taken and she was told the test revealed pneumonia.

Pneumonia is an infection of the lung in which a germ excites a reaction in the infected area. The invading germ is recognized by the immune system, which mounts a response consisting of attack cells called neutrophils. The interaction of the germ and these cells produces mucous that collect in the air sacs of the lung. The presence of this material in the infected area of the lung changes its consistency, which can be detected by an x-ray.

Mary was treated with an antibiotic and her primary physician did not encourage her to see a specialist, saying confidently, "You're young, it will go away."

Still her cough persisted and after another month she was referred to a lung specialist who ordered a CAT scan. A CAT scan uses x-rays and a computer program to produce a detailed cross-section image, providing the physician with information that cannot be gained from a standard x-ray.

The lung specialist concluded that the first antibiotic hadn't been effective and ordered a course of another drug. Mary continued to cough and another chest x-ray showed the condition to be unchanged. The pulmonologist then performed a procedure called a bronchoscopy. In this procedure, a thin, flexible fiberoptic tube or scope is passed through the nose, down the throat and into the windpipe, which leads to the lungs. Looking through the bronchoscope, the physician is able to see and examine the bronchial tubes and to obtain samples of mucous or tissue for study. After the procedure, Mary was told that swelling and irritation had been seen in her right lung, which the primary care physician had thought was due to the pneumonia.

Samples of mucous called "bronchial washings" were sent to a lab for study. These samples did not reveal evidence of infection and Mary was told that in time she should improve. Still coughing after a total of eight months, she decided to see yet another physician and she found me.

Mary and her family were clearly frustrated. She had had multiple doctor visits, multiple x-rays, and an uncomfortable procedure without the doctors being able to come to a clear understanding or diagnosis of her condition. None of the medications had been effective. At the time of her appointment with me she was taking a narcotic cough suppressant, which gave her a few hours of relief but had the side effect of making her drowsy and sluggish

"I can't live like this," she said plaintively. I totally understood how she must be feeling.

When I see a patient who has been evaluated by other physicians I ask the individual to start by describing their illness from its onset. I feel this is the only way to be objective and helps me hear clues that may have been missed by others, though of course I also review information from former records. Through repetition of facts an important piece of information may emerge, not considered relevant earlier.

It would have been easy to start with the diagnosis of pneumonia that the other doctors had made, but in listening to Mary's history of her illness I began to question whether she had ever had an infection. In infectious diseases, the typical signs that a physician looks for are fever, chills, and sweats. Mary had never experienced any of these. Her cough was deep and racking but had never produced phlegm. On two occasions, however, she had retched and noticed streaks of blood mixed with saliva when she expectorated. The medical term for this is hemoptysis.

As the months passed, Mary had also noted a decrease in her appetite and had lost six pounds. Recently she had experienced headaches, which she attributed to coughing all night.

The remainder of Mary's medical history was unremarkable: She had never been sick or hospitalized; her family's medical history was also without problems. During my physical examination of her, she coughed frequently, each time apologizing for the interruption. By listening to her chest with a stethoscope, I detected an area in the right lung in which the normal breath sounds were diminished. I knew this might be an indication of a blockage in one of the bronchial tubes.

When we breathe, air enters the nose and throat and passes into the windpipe. This large air tube divides into a main right and left bronchial tube responsible for the corresponding lung. The right lung has three divisions: Upper, middle, and lower sections called lobes. Mary's middle section was quiet. The air passing through the smaller and smaller bronchial channels ultimately enters air sacs called alveoli. If one of the air channels is blocked, the air in the air sacs beyond the blockage is absorbed and the sacs collapse. This condition is called atelectasis.

I reviewed Mary's chest x-rays and CAT scan. The air-filled lungs normally appear dark on a chest x-ray but the middle portion of Mary's right lung appeared white, indicating something solid was present. Her other physicians had interpreted this as pneumonia but the same finding can be atelectasis. The bronchial tube leading to the abnormal area appeared narrowed. This may have been what the other physician described as swelling.

Putting these findings together with what I had learned from her medical records and physical exam, I deduced that there was an obstruction in the bronchial tube leading to Mary's right middle lobe. A benign tumor, called a bronchial adenoma may be found in young people, producing a cough such as this girl experienced as well as the abnormalities that showed up in her x-rays. Such a growth may cause hemoptysis by breaking small blood vessels.

I could not explain, however, why this had not been seen by the other pulmonologist during the bronchoscopy but I noted that no sample of tissue or biopsy had been taken previously. Nearly three and a half months had passed since the procedure, so I wondered if a small lesion had been missed that might now be more obvious.

I also considered the possibility that Mary might have aspirated a foreign body. At the time that I saw Mary Kelly I had recently extracted a fruit pit from a patient's lungs whose x-rays showed similar findings. On another occasion I removed the cap of a ballpoint pen from a lung. Both objects had blocked the bronchial tubes producing atelectasis beyond the obstruction.

Unfortunately, another possibility was that Mary had lung cancer. Lung cancer, however, is usually a disease of middle age with only 2% of cases occurring before the age of 40. It would be extremely unlikely in Mary's case. The cancer mortality rate for people under the age of 29 is less than one per 100,000.

Lung cancer is one of the most common diagnoses that a lung specialist makes. There are nearly 200,000 new cases a year in the United States. It is also one of the most deadly malignancies with a five-year survival rate of only 14%. Mary was barely 22. The youngest patient I had ever diagnosed with lung cancer had been 39, and I had been practicing for many years before I met Mary. She had never smoked and the great majority of lung cancer cases, nearly 90 percent, occur in cigarette smokers. Both of her parents were non-smokers so she had not been exposed to secondhand smoke.

I always share the reasoning I've followed in making a diagnosis or deciding further steps to be taken, so after telling Mary and her family what I knew, I added that I wanted to repeat the bronchoscopy. I said that if my suspicion of a benign tumor was confirmed, it should be removed surgically. I wanted her to be prepared for what might be necessary after the bronchoscopy, and to help her focus on the possible resolution of her problem.

Because I feel it is extremely important that the patient participate in decision-making. I emphasized that though I was giving my opinion and recommendations, the final decision as to what would come next was up to her.

Mary and her family did not ask many questions, coming quickly to the main one, "When can it be done?"

"Soon," I said. "Very soon. I will perform the procedure myself."

The fiberoptic bronchoscope was developed by Japanese physicians and came into use in this country in 1969. I began my pulmonary fellowship in 1973 so that I had been performing this procedure for a very long time.

In my experience, many times a chest x-ray or CAT scan does not fully demonstrate the extent of a lung lesion. Mary's x-rays suggested a process localized in the middle portion of her right lung.

After participating in so many of these procedures over the years, it is difficult to recall in detail many specific cases. Mary Kelly's bronchoscopy is one of the exceptions. I remember clearly that as the bronchosope entered her windpipe or trachea, I saw immediately that at the lower end of this tube there appeared to be an inflammation. This redness extended from the lower end of the trachea into the right main bronchial tube and all of its branches including the middle lobe bronchus. On closer examination I suspected that this was more than the "irritation" the other pulmonologist had described. The lining of these tubes, which is called the mucosa, appeared infiltrated by a malignant tumor. This infiltration produced a lumpy appearance that severely distorted the normal passages and effectively blocked the middle lobe bronchial opening.

I was certain I was looking at a malignancy infiltrating Mary's right lung. Very few other illnesses can produce the extreme distortion and disruption of the normal bronchial tubes. I wondered if it could be any other malignancy besides lung cancer, perhaps a very rare tumor such as a sarcoma, which may occur in young people. I obtained several biopsies from the bronchial passages and took them personally to the laboratories where the tissue biopsies would be examined. I was unhappily sure of the answer I would be receiving in the next 48 hours.

I was hesitant to tell Mary just yet what I feared. At the same time I needed to prepare her for what I believed would be a diagnosis of malignancy and described to her the extent of the abnormality affecting her right lung. I said that it appeared to be caused by a growth or tumor. There was no need to go further. She was already ahead of me.

She immediately asked softly, "Could it be malignant?"

I told her that it was possible but very unusual at her age. We would have to wait for the pathologist's report to know. Mary appeared shaken but remained composed. I assured her I would review the slides with a pathologist the next day.

I make it a point to look at the slides of all of my biopsies. By doing so, I can see if my samples were adequate and at the same time obtain a first hand commentary from the pathologist. When I have an unusual or challenging case, I am often pacing the floor outside the pathology lab waiting for the slides to be ready. Mary's biopsy slides were in my hands the minute they were ready and I took them to one of the pathologists who placed them on a double-headed microscope so that we could look at the same time.

Usually I give the pathologist a short history of the case in question but this time I just said, "I have something unusual." He placed the slide under the microscope and began to examine the specimen. Without looking up he said, "It looks like large cell carcinoma…why so unusual?"

"Well, she's never smoked, and she's only 22."

"Are you sure? I've never heard of a case that young."

We went back together to look again at the slides. The pathologist said, "I need to make some special stains, but even without them, I am sure it is a large cell carcinoma."

In my heart I knew he was right. It was a very low moment for me.

The development of a cancer of the lung is a complex process that research has just begun to decipher. The end result of this process is damage to genetic material (DNA) resulting in the growth of a malignant cell. Malignancies grow and invade, unchecked by the body's inborn controls. Certain substances, such as tobacco smoke, have been shown to be carcinogens or promoters of the development of a cancer. Genetic factors are also thought to make some individuals more likely to develop cancer.

Mary Kelly had never smoked and had not been exposed to secondhand smoke so it was not clear to me how her malignancy had developed. I had to suspect one of the other known carcinogens, radon.

Radon is a gas released with the decay of radioactive material in soil. This gas may enter residential buildings through cracks in the foundation. The highest levels in homes have been found in basement areas, which may be poorly ventilated. Homes that are well insulated can trap radon in the house where it can become highly concentrated. When radon decays, tiny radioactive particles are produced which can be inhaled. The inhaled particles reach the lungs where they release radiation that can cause cancerous changes.

Studies of radon exposure in homes have concluded that it is a major cause of lung cancer and may account for 20,000 lung cancer deaths per year. Radon has been found in homes worldwide but high concentrations have been identified in Pennsylvania, New Jersey, and New York. Mary had lived with her family in a home in New Jersey all of her life; her bedroom was on the first floor. The house had never been checked for radon, the culprit I suspected.

The aggressiveness of a cancer is closely related to its rate of growth and tendency to spread or metastasize to lymph glands and other parts of the body. The most favorable malignancies grow slowly and do not spread so that they can be removed and possibly cured with surgery. Lung cancer is one of the least curable of all malignancies with only a 14% survival rate that is defined by living five years from the time of diagnosis. The reason for this poor outlook is that these cancers are typically discovered late in their course so that spread has already occurred.

Largely because of her age and the mind-set of her physicians that lung cancer cannot occur in someone so young, Mary Kelly's diagnosis had been delayed for eight months.

Once the diagnosis of a lung cancer is made, the next step is to screen the entire body for evidence of spread. This involves scanning the brain, abdominal cavity, and the skeleton, areas to which lung cancer has a tendency to spread. Large cell carcinoma is one of the four major types of lung cancer. Although not the fastest growing tumor, it may behave aggressively and involve lymph nodes or spread rapidly to other parts of the body. The extent of the tumor that I had seen at Mary's bronchoscopy indicated that she would require removal of the entire right lung (pneumonectomy) to remove the tumor completely.

At her age and without any other illness, I knew that she could tolerate this but first she would have to undergo the screening tests. If the cancer had already spread, there would be nothing gained by removing her lung.

After the pathologist confirmed his initial suspicion, I met with Mary and her family. Although I have now told hundreds of patients that they have lung cancer, it has not gotten any easier over time. I had never had to tell someone so young that they had a disease with so poor an outlook. I could not help but put myself in my patient's place and wonder how I would respond. Mary's life was just starting and I remembered ruefully her request for a cure before her upcoming marriage.

Mary's mother and fiancé were both with her when I told Mary gently that my suspicion of a tumor had been confirmed by the biopsy and that it was malignant, not benign. What caused it was unknown, I went on, but added that it could be treated, though it might mean removing her right lung.

All three listened intently as I went on. "She would first have screening tests of her entire body before surgery is undertaken. Then additional treatments such as radiation and chemotherapy might also be necessary."

Mary was trembling as she protested, "I don't understand…I've never smoked. The other doctors just told me to wait, I was so young, and it couldn't be anything serious…" Finally her protests stopped and she said, "I *knew* there was something really wrong."

I often tell medical students to listen carefully to patients because they themselves may perceive the nature of their illnesses and offer clues as to the correct diagnosis. After hearing a final diagnosis, it is not unusual for a patient to say that it was what they had suspected. I find this to be especially true in many patients with malignancy. This may be partly due to a fear of cancer that is heightened by a prolonged illness, but it is clear to me that many patients have insight into their illnesses.

While I was still with the little group, Mary's mother asked several questions about the prospective procedures, interspersed over and over again with a heartbroken query, "How could this happen? How could this happen?"

Her fiancé was unable to speak, tears filling his eyes. Taking his hand Mary spoke directly to me, "I don't think we should get married, do you?"

I answered indirectly, "Mary, you are going to need all of your strength for what is coming. Maybe someone from your church could better answer your question." The couple agreed. They would speak to the priest who was to perform the wedding ceremony.

Before our conversation was over I suggested to Mary's mother that she have their home tested for radon. It might provide the answer to her question of "how could this happen," and she agreed.

Several more minutes later I left Mary with her family to order her tests and to speak to a chest surgeon about the possible surgery.

The day after learning of the diagnosis she underwent a series of screening tests and as I ordered a CAT scan of the brain, I remembered Mary had complained of headaches. The scan showed two large masses in her brain that were probably metastases from her lung cancer.

I knew then that Mary's advanced disease could not be cured. The goal now was to extend her life as long as possible.

Radiation therapy to the brain tumors was started and Mary met with a cancer specialist who outlined a course of chemotherapy. Radiation therapy delivers intense heat that is directed at a specific site of malignancy while chemotherapy consists of administering toxic drugs. Both treatments kill cancer cells but do not completely eradicate a malignancy. In time the cancer recurs. There are also many side effects of these treatments such as hair loss, nausea, and a drop in blood count.

My physician involvement in Mary's care was almost over, though not my concern. But she was now under the care of others, so I did not see her for several weeks. Then one day I met her by accident as she was coming out of the hospital laboratory. She had finished her radiation therapy and had just had the first course of chemotherapy. She had lost her hair but I had no trouble recognizing her. She still had the same lovely, youthful face.

"Can we talk?" she asked.

"Sure," I said. "I want to hear how things are going."

We went up to my office where she told me the chemotherapy had made her ill but it had helped. She was improving, she said.

"But we're not getting married," she announced. "At least…not yet. I want to wait to see if I'll get better. I asked Dr. Jones, my oncologist, how long I have to live, but he wouldn't say." She looked straight into my eyes. "Do *you* know?"

This is the question that cancer patients are often afraid to ask, but not Mary.

I considered my response carefully. I knew too well that Mary's prognosis was more than poor, but didn't want to weaken her resolve by taking away the hope that she could get better. At the same time I wanted to tell her what she needed to know—whatever would help her decide how to live out the rest of her life.

"No one really knows," I began, "It depends on how you respond to the chemotherapy."

"I know that, but you have always been honest with me. I thought you might have some idea…" Her voice trailed off. She waited for my answer.

Should I tell her that only 50% of patients with large cell carcinoma already spread outside of the chest survive 12 months, even if treated with chemotherapy?

She was right. I had always told her the truth. She deserved an answer, for she had asked the question that even many of my much older patients could not bring themselves to ask.

I told her the medical statistics as non-threateningly as I could, emphasizing that these were only averages and that some patients live longer than 12 months.

"And some don't live that long?" she prodded.

I had to nod assent.

"Now," she said firmly, "I know what I have to do." She stood to leave.

Before I could ask what she meant, she reached the door, but turned back and said with great feeling, "*Thank you* for all that you have done."

The door closed and I fell silent. Had I done the right thing by answering her direct question directly? What did she mean, "I know what I have to do."?

We never had another conversation, Mary and I. Her malignancy proved resistant to treatment. She soon lapsed into a coma from the growth of tumor in her brain and spread of the cancer to her liver. Nearly three months to the day I had met her, I received a message from Dr. Jones. Mary was comatose, on life support in the intensive care unit.

I went immediately to the hospital's ICU to see her. She was unresponsive, her breathing supported by a respirator. I was struck once more by the youthfulness of her face, still quite lovely.

I reached for her hand and said aloud, "Mary, it's Dr. Adams." If she could hear, I wanted her to know that I was there.

Her mother was close by, and began to speak. "You were probably right about the radon, Doctor. You gave me the clue. I had the house tested and the results were very high." I saw the regret in her eyes. Unspoken were her words, "How could we have known?"

"Tomorrow was to have been her wedding day." She paused. "You know, after she asked you how much time she has left, she went to live with her fiancé. At least they've had a few weeks together."

I knew then what Mary meant when she had last spoken to me. How glad I was I'd told her the truth.

She died later that evening.

A few years later I saw a 34 year-old non-smoker who was also found to have large cell carcinoma of the lung at an advanced stage. His diagnosis had also been delayed and he died after six months despite chemotherapy. These two cases reinforced my assumption that when lung cancer occurs in the young, it is more aggressive than when it occurs in older patients.

A recent study, however, suggests that this is not true: The apparent increased aggressiveness is because the cancer is recognized too late for treatment to be effective. As in these two cases, delayed diagnosis may occur because with patients so young physicians often dismiss the possibility of lung cancer.

For a physician, the greatest joy is seeing a patient restored to good health. Fortunately, the majority of diseases that I treat are chronic respiratory conditions, which may never be cured, but can at least be controlled with appropriate medication and treatments. Unfortunately, there are many illnesses medicine does not cure.

Mary's "thank you" and others from patients with incurable, terminal diseases have taught me that a physician can provide comfort in many ways, even by just listening to what is said and responding honestly. When a patient dies it is natural for a doctor to feel that he has failed. I have never lost a patient without feeling inadequate, as if there was something else that I could have done. At such low points I try to think of what my patients, each in individual ways, have tried to tell me—that regardless of the outcome, I have made a difference, that they knew I was there.

3

For Love of Birds

o o o o o o o o o o o o o o o o o o o o o o o o o o o o o o o o o o o o

There is no recipe for living
That suits all cases

—*Carl Jung*

A physician is forever a student and an observer. The complexity of the human body and its myriad diseases provide never-ending medical challenges. To meet a challenge is exhilarating; to fail, humbling. A series of successes can often lead to thinking you have "seen it all." This is the trap that many physicians fall into and which may prevent their consideration of unusual illnesses. Whenever I begin to think that I have seen it all, I remember Katherine Cole.

It is more than 11 years since I met her, but I can still see Katherine as she entered my consultation room. She was accompanied by a friend, her "significant other," Robert Doherty, with whom she was then living. Katherine had given her age as 41 but appeared younger. What struck me then—and the impression remains in my memory—was that though youthful looking, her color and demeanor signaled a serious illness. When meeting a patient, doctors look for a spark of vitality—an indication of health that might show in the brightness of the eyes or skin tone. Katherine's skin was pale, her eyes dull.

She reported having severe headaches beginning about two months prior to our visit and had seen her primary physician for help. Her headaches were accompanied by nausea, changes in vision and a feeling of pressure on her neck—a tight, muscular sensation. The primary physician

29

referred her to a local neurologist, who arranged for an MRI to be taken of Katherine's brain; the image proved normal. An MRI produces very clear images of the body through the use of a large magnet, radio waves, and a computer. It has become the method of choice for looking at the brain.

She was told by the neurologist that her headaches were stress related, so a pain medication and a tranquilizer were prescribed, but Katherine felt worse while taking these prescriptions, experiencing both dizziness and ringing in her ears.

She then returned to her primary physician who performed a general examination, including a chest x-ray. The x-ray revealed a left lung mass that occupied a large part of her left lung. The physician gave Katherine a course of antibiotics, but her next chest x-ray did not show improvement. She was then advised to see a pulmonologist, and she was referred to me.

Katherine had never smoked and had always been in good health. I could not see anything from her medical history that suggested lung infection, although she had had a cold several months prior to the onset of her headaches. She reported no fevers, sweats, chills, and cough or chest pain.

"If I didn't have this horrible headache, I'd be fine," she said.

As I took Katherine's history, I thought of Mary Kelly and wondered if I was seeing another young woman who had never smoked but nevertheless developed lung cancer.

I asked Katherine a lot of questions, hoping to find some clues through knowing about her family, her travel, and even her pets. I learned she had three children, worked full time as a legal secretary and that her only medical condition was hay fever, which required very little treatment. She had a younger brother who had developed a benign lung tumor when he was only 31. She had never traveled outside of the United States and had lived in or near cities in the northeast all of her life. The family home in which she lived before marrying might have had asbestos in the basement but she didn't know for sure.

For eight months she had been living with Robert, who kept a pair of lovebirds in his home. Although they were Robert's pets, Katherine took care of them, changing the paper in their cage every day.

Her physical exam did not reveal much. She did not have any fever, weighed about 5 pounds under her usual weight, and although her chest sounds were quiet, I found no other abnormalities. I measured her lung capacity and oxygen level and found them normal.

Katherine's chest x-ray, however, was striking, especially in contrast to her seemingly normal medical history and physical exam. A large round mass, 10 centimeters in diameter, filled the upper third of her left lung. The interpreting radiologist told me he thought it was a lung cancer.

After the physical examination, I was at a loss. How did Katherine's headaches connect with her lung mass? Unlike the case of Mary Kelly, the MRI of Katherine's brain had been read as normal. Unless it had been misread, this would make spread of a lung cancer very unlikely. I asked her for the name of her neurologist so I could request a copy of the MRI to review.

At this point I wanted her to know what I was thinking, and we sat down to talk.

"I am not sure if your headaches are related to the shadow on your lung but I suspect that they are. The lung shadow could be a tumor, even a malignancy, but it could also be from an infection. In order to find out more I would like to look into your lung with an instrument called a bronchoscope that can take samples for analysis. Once we know what's causing the lung problem I think the source of the headaches will become clear."

Katherine agreed to have the bronchoscopy, saying, "I can't go on like this."

Since it was then Friday afternoon, the procedure was scheduled for the following Tuesday. She would go home and rest over the weekend.

With many illnesses, the manifestations of a disease may increase over time, providing the physician with more information and ultimately point him to a diagnosis. I did not suspect that the cause of Katherine's illness would appear so quickly.

The next morning Robert found that Katherine was hard to wake up. She seemed confused and complained of drowsiness, increased headache and neck pain. Robert called my answering service to report these worrisome symptoms. I suggested that they come to the hospital emergency room and I alerted the ER staff, asking one of our attending neurologists, David Lang, to see her after she was admitted.

After examining her, Dr. Lang called me. "I don't know what's going on in her lung, but her neck is stiff and she has signs of meningitis. I think she needs a spinal tap."

Meningitis is an infection of the membranes that cover the brain and spinal cord. Patients with this disease often complain of a stiff neck. Many types of infections may cause meningitis, so to pinpoint the cause of the disease and to confirm the diagnosis, a sample of spinal fluid must be obtained and analyzed.

A spinal tap or lumbar puncture is one of the first procedures that a medical student learns and I still remember my first. The patient lies on one side in the fetal position to best expose the lower back. A local anesthetic similar to Novocain is injected into the skin between two bones or vertebrae and a long spinal needle is inserted. There is a slight popping sound as the needle enters the spinal column. To a medical student there is nothing better than seeing those first drops of spinal fluid fall from the hub of the needle for this tells you that you are in. A sample of the fluid is collected and analyzed.

Spinal fluid is normally crystal clear but Katherine's looked a little cloudy. The cloudiness was due to an increased number of white blood cells in the fluid. These cells are infection fighters and attack the invading organism, trying to neutralize it. In a small laboratory off the emergency room, a neurology resident prepared a slide of the spinal fluid and looked at it under a microscope, hoping to identify the source of the infection. Special stains or other chemicals are often used to highlight the microscopic germs for identification. One of these preparations mixes India ink with the spinal fluid. As the resident scanned Katherine's India ink slide, her eyes lit up and she alerted Dr. Lang who came in to look. I received another call.

"We have a diagnosis. It's cryptococcosis."

What the resident and attending neurologists had seen in the India ink preparation were many round yeast forms, each with a very clear, bright outer capsule. The contrast of the India ink makes them stand out, like little glowing globes in a sea of blackness. This is the characteristic appearance of a fungus or yeast known as cryptococcus neoformans. A sample of Katherine's spinal fluid was also placed in an agar dish and incubated at body temperature in order to culture organisms. After 48 hours a white mold appeared in the agar dish and this was also identified as cryptococcus. Both her blood and spinal fluid were found to contain a very high quantity of a protein substance called cryptococcal antigen, derived from this fungus.

The diagnosis of meningitis due to cryptococcus infection had been confirmed but many questions remained to be answered. How had she acquired this rare infection? I had seen cases of cryptococcus only in patients with lowered immunity due to AIDS or cancer. Did Katherine have an HIV infection and AIDS or an occult malignancy? Was the mass on her x-ray also due to the same fungus? How should she be treated?

Cryptococcus neoformans occurs in nature and has been found in soil samples from around the world in areas frequented by birds, especially chickens and pigeons. It may be found in rotting vegetation and in bird guano. Birds do not become sick from cryptococcus but do harbor the fungus in their digestive tracts. It is thought that birds acquire the germ by eating contaminated vegetation. Human infection occurs through inhalation of the fungus into the respiratory tract. From there, the germ multiplies and may enter the bloodstream and travel to other organs such as the brain. Cryptococcus has a tendency to localize in the brain where it appears to grow more easily than in other parts of the body.

It was now clear to me that Katherine had inhaled tiny yeast forms into her lungs that had spread through her bloodstream to her brain where they multiplied and caused meningitis. The mass in her lung was most likely the site of the original lung infection but I had never seen or read of such a large mass from this fungal infection.

Not long after speaking to Dr. Lang I thought of Robert's lovebirds. Lovebirds are the smallest members of the parrot family. I knew of the association of cryptococcus with pigeons but was not sure if other birds can also be implicated in causing this infection.

Katherine had already been told about the diagnosis by Dr. Lang, and had been admitted to the hospital where I saw her the next day. I asked her to describe how she took care of the birds. She saw where my question was leading.

"Is that how you think I got this crypto whatever-it-is? I never liked those birds. All they do is poop!" That comment gave us both a laugh, which we needed.

She described changing the newspaper in the bottom of their cage every day, crumbling it and throwing it into the trash.

"Sometimes I hold my breath, especially when there's a cloud of dust."

I told her I wasn't sure if this was the source and asked if she lived or worked near pigeons, chickens, or other birds.

"Just the ones in our living room and they're not going to be there much longer." (I later heard that Robert removed the birds that night.)

I explained to Katherine the need to order an HIV test. "If you have a weakened immune system, it might explain how this germ took hold."

She didn't hesitate about having the blood test. I knew that the great majority of patients with cryptococcosis have other diseases that may have damaged their immune systems, the most common being AIDS. I had only seen the disease before in a few AIDS patients and in one man with Hodgkin's disease, a form of cancer of the lymph glands. I had read case reports describing the disease in patients who had received organ transplants and were on anti-rejection medications, but I had never seen a case in a patient with normal immunity.

Happily, Katherine's HIV test proved to be negative.

When physicians are confronted with extraordinary diseases rarely encountered, they must then refresh their memories with information learned in early medical training. I went deeply into my library of textbooks and journals to learn more about cryptococcosis.

The journal articles confirmed that other birds had been connected with this rare infection. I found one report of a patient with a pet cockatoo who developed cryptococcal meningitis but noted that he was taking medications to prevent rejection of a kidney transplant. Cryptococcus was found in the cockatoo's droppings and it was identical to the fungus isolated from the patient.

I also found that most lung masses from this disease were smaller than Katherine's, measuring usually four centimeters in diameter or less. I knew that there was an association with cancer and cryptococcosis and wondered if she was suffering from two separate diseases.

I met with Katherine and Robert again and shared what I had learned. I told them I thought it was necessary to proceed with the bronchoscopy to be sure that the lung mass wasn't a lung cancer or a site of lymphoma. She agreed and I scheduled the procedure for the next day.

The only abnormality I saw through the bronchoscope was some mild redness in the area of the bronchial tubes leading to the left upper lung. The biopsies and washings I obtained, however, were very abnormal. I reviewed the slides with one of our pathologists. The biopsy samples were striking, showing numerous yeast forms within the tissue of the lung. There was nothing else to suggest malignancy or another infection. Katherine's lung mass was also due to the same fungal infection that had caused her meningitis. I now knew that with a negative HIV test, my patient had an excellent chance of a complete recovery.

From the moment that Dr. Lang called to report finding cryptococcus, I knew I would need help in treating this infection and asked one of our infectious disease specialists, Dr. Anthony Martins, to consult. On the night of Katherine's admission, Dr. Martins initiated treatment with two anti-fungal medications, amphotericin and 5-fluocytosine. He would continue to follow Katherine's case closely with me for several years.

Amphotericin can be given only by intravenous infusion, and is often called "ampho-terrible" because of its numerous side effects. A small test dose is given on the first day and the dosage gradually increased. Some of the most common side effects are chills, fever, nausea, vomiting and loss of appetite. The more serious side effects include seizures, irregular heartbeat, kidney failure, internal bleeding, and liver dysfunction. Unfortunately it is the mainstay of anti-fungal treatment and Katherine would receive 42 days of infusions of amphotericin before leaving the hospital. The second anti-fungal drug is given by mouth and commonly causes nausea and at times vomiting.

I saw Katherine each morning. Many days I could see that she was ill from these potent drugs but she never voiced any objection to her treatment, asking only how long it would be necessary to keep on with the treatment.

"How will you know when I can go home?" was her only question.

I explained what Dr. Martins had advised.

"We will follow your blood level of cryptococcal antigen, continue your x-rays and repeat a spinal tap in two weeks to find out if the fungus has disappeared from your spinal fluid. If the results show improvement, then another anti-fungal pill will be substituted for the amphotericin and then you can leave the hospital."

Katherine's infection proved so stubborn she was hospitalized for six weeks. Her headaches and neck pain disappeared slowly. Her second spinal tap showed no evidence of yeast forms. She was greatly relieved after hearing the results, but I had to tell her, "You will have to stay on the anti-fungal pills for as long as the cryptococcal antigen remains positive, possibly a year or more."

The prospect of a long duration of treatment didn't seem to bother her. "As long as I don't have to take the amphotericin, I won't mind."

To see a patient daily who is recovering from a serious illness can be an enriching experience. I look each day on my rounds for signs that reflect a return to well-being—brightness of the eyes, skin tone, posture, and speech quality. Katherine's physical appearance improved and though she was thin and seemed almost frail, she had a high tolerance for pain and discomfort as well as a good sense of humor. Her complaints were few and never trivial, but she was often anxious and required frequent reassurance that she was improving and would recover completely.

After six weeks of treatment Katherine's condition improved significantly. Her cryptococcal antigen blood level was still very elevated but had started to decline and her chest x-rays showed a slight decrease in the size of the lung mass. Both Dr. Martins and I met with Katherine on the day of her discharge to discuss the treatment plan. She would see both of us once a month and have a blood test and chest x-ray at the time of her visits. Her anti-fungal medication was to consist of two oral medications to be continued until the cryptococcal antigen could no longer be detected.

It might take a year—possibly two—but a complete cure was likely, we told her. I remember that Katherine's appearance on the day of her discharge was completely different from the day she entered my office. Her eyes were bright and she smiled frequently, clearly relieved to be going home, not needing any more amphotericin treatment.

During the first year I noticed that Robert no longer accompanied her to office visits and one day she left me a new address and said, "Robert and I are no longer together." She did not volunteer more information and I didn't ask for any.

I did not foresee then that Katherine would still be under my care seven years later. Throughout this long convalescence she never missed an appointment nor failed to take her medication. At each of her office visits I took a new chest x-ray and measured the size of the left lung mass. During the first two years, both the size of the mass and the cryptococcal blood level decreased steadily. Katherine was tolerating the oral medications and was bolstered by the reports of gradual improvement in her laboratory studies.

There were anxious moments. On a visit nearly one year after discharge Katherine said, "I think it's back. My neck hurts and I have ringing in my ears." After an exam and an x-ray I told her that all indicators pointed to improvement and that a relapse was not likely.

"Your pain seems to radiate from your shoulder. Let's look for another explanation."

An MRI of her shoulder was taken which revealed a tendon tear. With physical therapy, her pain disappeared. The ringing in her ears was caused by one of her medications; after the dosage was reduced, it disappeared.

Between the third and fourth years after discharge from the hospital, Katherine's cryptococcal antigen and chest x-ray remained about the same. The mass had decreased from 10 to 2.5 centimeters, but then stopped shrinking. Despite reassurance from both Dr. Martins and me, I could sense with each visit that Katherine's anxiety was increasing. She had tolerated the anti-fungal medications but had experienced annoying side effects such as nausea. She also had to be careful to avoid interactions of these medications with other drugs. At the end of one of her visits she asked bleakly, "Will I ever be able to stop these drugs without the disease coming back?"

The infectious disease consultant and I spoke frequently. Towards the end of the fourth year, he said, "She may have to have that lung mass removed since there may be fungal forms within it that the antibiotics can't reach."

Lung masses that develop from fungal infections often harbor germs for long periods of time. Once again, I looked into the medical literature for guidance. I found several reports of similar cases in which a cure was achieved only after the lung mass was removed surgically. I knew then there would have to be a major operation.

The procedure is called a thoracotomy. Chest surgeons perform it frequently for the exploration and removal of many different lung lesions. In order to enter the chest the surgeon must make a long incision along the plane of the ribs, beginning at about the tip of the shoulder blade and ending just beneath the beginning of the breast. The ribs are then spread to allow access to the chest cavity. With a thoracotomy, patients typically experience severe pain post-operatively and require several weeks for recuperation.

In the last several years, however, a less invasive procedure called a "video-guided thoracoscopic resection" has been used in place of a thoracotomy in certain patients. The new procedure resembles the laparoscopic operations, sometimes called "band aid surgery," that have been used for abdominal surgery. I wondered if Katherine's fungal mass could be removed with the less traumatic video-guided procedure.

Dr. Martins and I explained the situation to Katherine. It was hard news to give, but I had to tell her our best opinion.

"We can go on with the anti-fungal medications, hoping that they will work, but it has been a long time since your blood test and x-ray have changed. We think that the lung mass should be removed. Judging by the experience of other patients, this procedure should allow you to stop the anti-fungal medications."

I saw concern on Katherine's face but she had trusted us for a long time. She didn't waver now.

"If you think that this surgery will do it, let's go ahead."

I arranged for her to meet with one of the hospital's chest surgeons who then scheduled the procedure. He would attempt to remove the mass with the video procedure and if it proved impossible, then perform a thoracotomy.

In the operating room the surgeon made three small incisions in the left side of Katherine's chest and introduced an instrument called a thoracoscope. The thoracoscope is a long, rigid tube the surgeon can look through and connect to a video camera. The top or apex of Katherine's lung was found to be stuck to the undersurface of the ribs. This is common in fungal and tuberculous infections of the lung. The surgeon freed the lung with his instruments but then found that the portion needing removal was too big for the video-guided approach. The thoracoscope was withdrawn and the thoracotomy performed. A large portion of the upper section or lobe of the left lung was removed and sent to pathology.

In the laboratory, the pathologist cut through the specimen exposing a round nodule of 2.5 centimeters containing a center of white, cheesy material. Katherine had received nearly four and a half years of anti-fungal treatment but on examining the material under the microscope the pathologist still found numerous yeast forms typical of cryptococcus. In another lab, a portion of the specimen was placed in an incubator. After 48 hours, a white mold was cultured, again identified as cryptococcus. Dr. Martins had been right; the fungus had survived four and a half years of treatment by hiding in an area of the lung where the anti-fungal medications could not reach. The decision to remove the mass had been the correct one.

Katherine's age and general good health allowed her to recover from the surgery. Although experiencing considerable pain and discomfort she again demonstrated the strength and resolve to be well. The difficult dissection of her lung required a two-week stay in the hospital but on hearing the news of the pathologist's report, her spirits lifted. "That means I could have taken the medications for ten or twenty years and the fungus would still be there. I knew this was the right decision."

One month after surgery, Katherine's cryptococcal antigen had fallen by half and her anti-fungal medications were stopped. She also stopped all painkillers and felt well. In the next twelve months, her blood level of cryptococcal antigen fell again by half; after another year it was nearly undetectable. She continued to see me once a year, and on each visit another x-ray was taken. Other than the signs of having had surgery, her x-rays remained clear. With each good report and mention of a cure in sight, she sighed with relief.

Seven and a half years after our first meeting we had our last visit. Katherine radiated good health, looking not a day older than when we had first met. She had changed jobs and appeared happy. The final chest x-ray was again clear. "Your blood and x-ray have been clear for more than three years since your surgery. There's no doubt in my mind that you are completely cured." We were both beaming.

"Say it again! Am I really cured? Does that mean you're discharging me?"

I anticipated her next question. "The truth is that you don't need a lung specialist anymore and that's a good thing. I'm going to miss you Katherine. You've been a wonderful patient, and I've appreciated knowing you. I only wish your insurance company would cover visits to a specialist for an inactive disease.

"I know it sounds strange but insurance approval for continued visits would only be granted if you become sick again and I don't believe that is going to happen. If you need me for anything, though, I'll be here."

We both smiled, she thanked me warmly, and we said good-bye.

For a physician there is no greater pleasure that seeing a patient restored to good health. To witness a full recovery from a life-threatening illness that requires challenging decision-making is exhilarating and satisfying. Each case is a learning process and Katherine's had provided me with a tremendous amount of knowledge and experience as well as one very important lesson. No matter how long you practice medicine, you have never seen it all.

4

Never Give Up

"Never give in. Never give in. Never give in"

—*Winston Churchill*

Kevin O'Connor was my patient and my friend for eighteen years. Something about his vibrant personality coupled with his will to live have left him with a special place in my heart. We were the same age, grew up in the same area, were rabid sports fans and we bonded from the moment I met him in spite of the fact that we supported rival teams! This is the third book in which I find myself inspired to write about him.

Kevin had an engaging sense of humor, often self-deprecating. On the surface, he appeared not to take life too seriously but, as I learned, he had the strongest will to survive of any patient I have ever encountered.

Kevin was initially referred to me because of a severe cough. During his first visit I asked questions about his lifestyle and any past medical problems. He revealed that he had had frequent bouts of chest infections since childhood, always diagnosed as bronchitis. He started smoking in his early teens and now at 36, was still smoking one to two packs of cigarettes a day. As a teenager he ran track competitively and now as an adult jogged two miles once or twice a week "when I have the wind."

At least twice a year he developed a severe cough, "like fits," he described them. During these infections he coughed up green phlegm and experienced shortness of breath. A week before our first visit, he had a shortness of breath he said felt like "hyperventilation." He had also felt pain over his left chest causing his internist to order a chest x-ray, which he

42

had brought to show me. The day before the pains started he had been lifting heavy boxes, but the chest pain didn't start until the following day.

Kevin's medical history was unremarkable except for his chest problems. He had been "allergic to everything as a child," he said, but had "outgrown" this problem. There was no history of lung disease in his family. Though Kevin had managed several restaurants, he had never been exposed to noxious chemicals or fumes. He drank socially but did not engage in any substance abuse.

I performed a physical examination and found that Kevin's breathing sounds were much quieter than normal. A decrease in the loudness of breath sounds may be found in a number of diseases but may also signal emphysema.

The lung contains millions of tiny air sacs or alveoli that exchange oxygen and carbon dioxide with the blood. In emphysema, the walls between these air sacs are destroyed producing larger cyst-like spaces in which air stagnates and is not refreshed. Occasionally these cysts, called bullae, may be very large. The type of emphysema in which large cysts occur is referred to as *bullous*. The loss of the air sacs also decreases the natural elasticity of the lungs. It is the elastic property of the lung that gives it the ability to snap back and exhale air after it is inhaled. This loss of elasticity contributes to difficulty exhaling, further trapping air in the cyst-like spaces. This trapped air produces over-inflation, which compresses undamaged portions of the lungs, interfering with the normal exchange of oxygen and carbon dioxide in healthy areas.

The most common cause of emphysema is cigarette smoking and this appeared to be the cause of Kevin's disease. When lungs are exposed to the irritation of cigarette smoke, the body responds by sending immune cells, called macrophages, to the site of irritation. These cells produce an enzyme, called *elastase* that destroys the walls of the air sacs, resulting in emphysema. This destructive enzyme is normally held in check by inhibiting or neutralizing substances, but cigarette smoke stops their function, allowing elastase to go unchecked and destroy lung tissue.

Kevin had had numerous bouts of infection involving the bronchial tubes. These bouts of bronchitis had further inflamed the air passages or bronchial tubes of his lungs. Numerous studies have demonstrated that smokers develop several times the number of chest infections as non-smokers because the contents of cigarette smoke interferes with the delicate defense mechanisms built into the lining of the bronchial tubes. This lining is called the *mucosa* and consists of several layers of tissue designed to protect and nourish the airways of the lung. The surface layer consists of a blanket of microscopic wands called *cilia* that sweep back and forth, trapping and ejecting germs and foreign material. In cigarette smokers, the cilia are damaged or obliterated so that infecting organisms have a greater opportunity to invade and produce infection.

After obtaining Kevin's medical history and giving him a physical examination, I concluded that cigarette smoking had produced both bronchitis and emphysema in this young man, but I did not realize the extent of his disease until I looked at his chest x-ray.

The divisions of the lungs are called lobes. The right lung consists of an upper, middle, and lower lobe and the left lung has an upper and lower division. Kevin's x-ray revealed that large cysts or bullae had replaced both upper lobes. I could not see any normal lung in these areas. Smaller cysts were also visible in the lower lobes. I ordered breathing tests, amazed that he was able to continue to run and to exercise.

Despite the massive bullae, Kevin's biggest and deepest breath, which is called the *vital capacity,* was a surprising 76 per cent of what is normal for his age, height, weight, and sex (normal range is 80–100) and his blood oxygen level was near normal. These facts and the rest of the breathing study told me that Kevin's middle and lower lobes functioned well, despite the compression of the bullae. I thought that if Kevin would stop smoking and avoid infection, he could lead a normal life.

We sat down to go over the results of his tests and I emphasized the need for him to stop smoking immediately. As a former smoker, I know firsthand the strength of nicotine addiction so that when I work with patients who need to stop, I tell them my own experience and that over many years of working with patients, I've learned that motivation is the key to stopping. I offered motivation for Kevin by telling him that he and he alone would determine the quality of his life.

"You can continue to smoke and suffer more and more damage. This will lead to a drop in your oxygen level so that within five, maybe ten years, you will be so short of breath that getting dressed in the morning or taking a shower will be difficult. You won't even be 50 years old."

Although Kevin recognized the seriousness of the situation he grinned his irrepressible grin and said, "Are you telling me I won't be able to have sex?"

I laughed, "Yes, among other things."

As our discussion continued I learned that Kevin was divorced but was seeing someone new. My message about sex hit home; he agreed to stop smoking, so I prescribed a nicotine chewing gum and told him to increase his exercise routine.

After six weeks Kevin came for another visit and reported that he was feeling much better, was running a mile and a half a day and had resolved never to resume smoking. During the next year I saw him only once for a new chest infection.

Just a little more than a year later, Kevin returned. He had changed jobs and had been smoking again for several months. Maybe the stress of the new job had gotten to him, I thought to myself.

He was having low-grade fevers and a chill, lost 16 pounds, had swelling in his ankles, pains in his joints and was vomiting frequently. His fingernails had become curved or "clubbed." Clubbing of the nails may occur along with many types of lung and heart disease although the exact cause is unknown.

I ordered a new chest x-ray and was alarmed at the results. A huge 8x10 centimeter mass in the middle of Kevin's right lung was visible. It hadn't been present on his x-ray one year earlier. I discussed the findings with a staff radiologist who had also seen the x-ray. We both felt that one of Kevin's large cysts had probably become infected and that the large mass represented infected fluid. Lung cancer seemed less likely in view of the massiveness of the growth in a relatively short time.

I told Kevin the results and that I needed to place him on antibiotics to treat the infection. He left my office with a prescription but called me the next day to report a temperature of 103 degrees. I didn't hesitate.

"You need to be in the hospital to receive antibiotics intravenously so they can reach the site of your infection in full strength. The pills are not working." Kevin was admitted that night and received two powerful anti-biotics through a vein.

After ten days on these medications, the next x-ray had not improved and I ordered a chest CAT scan. The results were disturbing. Kevin's mass was more solid than what might be expected from infected fluid within a cyst. I now questioned our original diagnosis of an infected cyst. Kevin's cigarette smoking had produced emphysema and bronchitis; I now sus-pected lung cancer as well.

I told Kevin the CAT scan results and the need to perform a bronchos-copy. Kevin asked directly, "Do you think I have cancer?"

"It looks suspicious, especially since the antibiotics aren't working but we won't know until we have a biopsy." A bronchoscopy was scheduled for the next morning.

My late wife Laurie, an RN, was assisting me with bronchoscopies in those days. She was my secret weapon in getting patients to relax because she had a tremendous empathy with my patients. After I introduced her as my wife, patients would invariably begin to chat with her, pleased that the two of us worked together as a team. As in many procedures, considerable anxiety mounts with anticipation of what is about to occur during the bronchoscopy, as well as fear of what might be found.

Kevin and Laurie connected immediately and he made her laugh. He kidded her, saying "I hope he pays you well," and "He can at least take you out to dinner after this," and "I'm getting the attention of two for the price of one."

While they laughed and talked, Kevin relaxed, distracted by his own levity. After administering a sedative and local anesthetic I passed the bronchoscope into Kevin's lungs. On examining the bronchial openings to his right lower lobe I found that two channels were compressed. I couldn't see a growth within the tubes but there seemed to be pressure on these tubes from a surrounding mass. I rinsed the areas with a saline solution and submitted the washings to the pathology department.

The next day I looked at the slides with our pathologist.

"Malignancy looks more than likely, but I can't say for sure. We need a larger sample."

I went to Kevin's room to tell him the results. He was willing to undergo the procedure again but I told him I had another idea.

"The better approach may be from the outside of your chest since the openings were closed from within. I would like to schedule a needle biopsy."

I explained that in this technique a radiologist pinpoints the area to be sampled by using the CAT scanner. A local anesthetic is injected into the skin and a thin needle is passed through into the lung and the mass. Material from the mass is aspirated back into a syringe. Kevin was disappointed to hear that Laurie did not assist in this procedure but quickly agreed anyway.

The next day a radiologist positioned Kevin in the CAT scanner and obtained an exact location and depth to which he would pass a long, thin needle. He performed two "passes" and obtained samples from the center of the mass. This time the result was definitive. Kevin's mass was a lung cancer that the pathologist said was undifferentiated. This term describes a fast growing malignancy, which explained how Kevin's mass had reached huge proportions in less than a year. I knew the only treatment that could remove the cancer was through surgery. Could he tolerate such a procedure with his coexisting emphysema? Had his rapidly growing tumor already spread to other areas of his body as in Mary Kelly's case?

I told Kevin about the diagnosis, about possible surgery and about my reservations because of potential complications. He remained composed, but this time he didn't joke. He said emphatically, "I want this thing removed."

I outlined my plan.

"We will scan your entire body to see if the cancer has spread, then repeat breathing tests to be sure you still have a good lung capacity and can tolerate removal of part of your right lung. I also want to do a special scan of your lungs to see which areas are healthy and functioning, and which sections are permanently damaged. If the healthy areas are close to the cancer, you may not be able to afford their removal. If you pass all these preliminary tests, I will call in a chest surgeon and an oncologist."

Kevin's brain and abdomen CAT scans proved normal. A bone scan performed with a radioactive tracer did not reveal malignancy but did explain why Kevin had developed clubbing of his nails and swollen ankles. Lung cancers are known to be capable of manufacturing hormonal substances. One of these hormones that may be produced is growth hormone normally active early in life, stimulating skeletal growth. When this substance enters the blood stream of a mature adult, it further stimulates bone reaction, producing Kevin's finger and joint symptoms that together are known as *hypertrophic osteoarthopathy*.

Kevin also underwent a lung scan similar to that used in the diagnosis of a pulmonary embolus in which a radioactive isotope or tracer is injected and inhaled. By following the radioactive material through these separate routes into Kevin's lungs, the radiologist was able to tell me which areas were functioning and which was permanently damaged. The results were encouraging to me. The site of Kevin's malignancy and the area that would have to be removed was his right lower lobe. The scan showed that this lobe accounted for only 20 percent of Kevin's total breathing capacity, which is significantly less than the normal of 33 percent. Based on this information and Kevin's pulmonary function tests, I concluded that he could afford to have the right lower lobe removed and still have enough lung function to lead an active life. However, Kevin would have difficulty breathing if his entire right lung had to be removed due to extension of the tumor into other lobes.

I presented my opinion to the chest surgeon with whom I worked most frequently. He examined Kevin and reviewed his x-rays and scans but came to a different conclusion.

"I may not be able to remove the mass without removing his entire right lung and if I do, I think his left lung may collapse. He may end up on a respirator. I think he's inoperable."

We discussed our disparate views back and forth but did not come to a consensus. The surgeon felt he had no choice but to tell Kevin his opinion and suggested that he see an oncologist.

Within a few hours Kevin heard more bad news. The oncologist agreed with the surgeon and told Kevin that he recommended chemotherapy to treat the rapidly growing cancer. He also predicted that at best he had six months to live.

Despite the opinions from both consultants I still felt strongly that Kevin could have surgery and survive. I went to his room to tell him my divergent opinion.

Kevin was angry when I got there and ready to beat the odds. I told him that I didn't agree with the surgeon or the oncologist.

"The surgeon says I'm inoperable and the oncologist says I have six months! I think you're right and they're wrong. You know what? I'm going to come back here in six months and piss on both their desks! So what's the next step—what do we do now?"

I was happy to see Kevin willing to do battle. I had a plan but it would take a great deal of strength and resolve on his part.

"We're going to get a second surgical opinion from Dr. Nael Martini at Memorial-Sloan Kettering. He and I have met at conferences and he strikes me as a surgeon with a lot of experience and imagination. It's the combination we need."

Kevin was raring to go.

"I like him already, when can I see him?"

I called Dr. Martini the next day and told him that I had a challenging case and needed his help. "Kevin is a 38-year-old smoker with bullous emphysema and recently diagnosed lung cancer. My studies show that he's a surgical candidate but my surgical consultant feels that he's inoperable. I'd like to have your opinion."

Dr. Martini agreed to see him, so I sent Kevin to his appointment with a huge stack of records and scans under his arm. A few days later I received a call from Dr. Martini.

"I think you're right about surgery and it is this young fellow's only chance at survival, but first I have to operate on his left lung to improve his chances."

I heard from Kevin shortly after this conversation, thanking me for sending him to Memorial. I asked him if he knew he was going to have two operations.

"Sure. It's going to be a piece of cake. They open one side, fix it, then a week later, they open the other side and take out the cancer. I don't know how to thank you. Not many doctors would send someone to another hospital other than their own."

I asked him to call me after each surgery, though I would also be receiving updates from Dr. Martini as well.

Kevin was admitted to Memorial the next day and the following morning Dr. Martini performed a left thoracotomy. On opening his chest, the surgeon found four large bullae, occupying 90% of the left upper lobe. These cysts were then excised and the left lower lobe was then explored. Smaller cysts were found and these were also removed. By performing this procedure, the healthy lung tissue in Kevin's left lung was freed of the compression of these cysts, improving his breathing capacity. I heard from Kevin the next day and from the slow pattern of his speech I could tell he was full of pain medication, though he spoke jokingly.

"One down and one to go, if I'm still here next week."

I knew he was all right since his sense of humor was intact and encouraged him to get some rest to be ready for the next procedure.

One week later, Dr. Martini performed a right thoracotomy. Large bullae were found in the right upper lobe and these were removed first. The tumor mass in the right lower lobe was then completely removed with the entire lobe and several lymph glands. Exploration of and removal of lymph glands is a standard procedure in cancer surgery. The lymph glands are part of the body's immune system and regional glands drain their respective areas. If Kevin's lung cancer had spread, the first area to become involved would have been the lymph glands draining the region of his right lower lobe. Kevin's pathology report was encouraging. All of the lymph glands that were removed were free of cancer.

Less than three weeks after entering Memorial, Kevin was discharged after having two major operations. He had tolerated both operations well though requiring pain medication for a while. His mood was upbeat.

"Remember what I'm coming back to do on a certain surgeon's desk? I'll let you know when it's time."

Dr. Martini and I both thought he had a good chance of survival and that the major treatment for his malignancy was behind him. We had no idea of what was coming.

One month after leaving Memorial Kevin made an appointment with me in my office. I had expected him to walk in with a smile on his face but when I saw his serious expression I knew something was wrong. He told me he had developed headaches and that his vision was "off." I asked him to describe what he meant.

"I see flashing lights before my eyes, even when I close them. I can't read even a newspaper or the numbers on my alarm clock."

I knew only too well that lung cancer commonly spreads to the brain and immediately ordered a brain CAT scan and arranged for Kevin to see a neurologist.

Kevin reminded me that his brain study before surgery had been normal.

"Can it really spread that fast?" he asked with disbelief.

"Not usually," I responded. I could hardly believe it myself.

Kevin's brain CAT scan showed dramatic changes. Nerve fibers that control vision originate in a portion of the brain called the occipital lobe. Kevin's scan showed a cluster of three round masses in his right occipital lobe with surrounding swelling of the brain tissue. The radiologists thought it showed carcinoma that had spread from the lung cancer. A neurosurgeon and a radiation oncologist were also consulted and a plan was formed. Kevin would undergo radiation therapy to the brain followed by a repeat CAT scan. If the lesions did not respond, he would then undergo brain surgery to remove the mass.

I saw Kevin after the neurosurgeon left and he was full of confidence.

"I can beat this, Frank, even if they have to make a hole in my head."

Radiation damages the genetic material in cancer cells causing them to die or reduce their growth. It is usually given in small doses over an extended period of time in order to allow surrounding normal cells to repair themselves. Each treatment must be strong enough to kill the cancer cell while avoiding permanent damage to normal structures. Unfortunately, this goal is not always met and the tissues in the path of the x-ray beam may be affected. Cancers vary greatly in their response to radiation treatments. Some cancer cells are "sensitive" or easily killed by radiation while others are "resistant" and do not respond. The location and size of a malignancy may be an important factor in determining the success or failure of radiation therapy. This relates to the amount of radiation that can be delivered to the core of a cancer mass.

Kevin received a course of radiation to the brain over a ten-day period but a repeat CAT scan did not show shrinkage of the lesion. Instead, the mass appeared more cystic and filled with fluid. The neurosurgeon attempted to reach the lesion by making a burr hole in the back of Kevin's skull but this was unsuccessful. He then performed a larger procedure called a craniotomy in which a piece of the skull is removed, permitting wider exposure of the brain. Kevin's mass was localized and the cyst was drained of fluid and the whole lesion removed.

I reviewed the results with one of the hospital's radiologists and was surprised to hear that, "There's no cancer in this mass, just the wall of a cyst. Either the cancer was completely eradicated by the radiation or this was an abscess from the start. Unfortunately we will never know for sure."

I wondered whether the mass could really have been an abscess in the first place since Kevin had not received any antibiotic therapy and no germs were recovered from the specimen. I concluded that Kevin's cancer was very sensitive to radiation therapy though I knew of rare reports of lung cancers cured with radiation therapy. Kevin's neurosurgeon questioned my theory and he concluded that the lesion had been an abscess all along. I didn't know then that the sensitivity of Kevin's cancer to radiation would be soon be demonstrated once more.

Throughout the period that Kevin was receiving the brain radiation and recovering from the craniotomy, a series of routine chest x-rays were taken over a three-month period. I reviewed each one and had gone to the x-ray department to see the latest x-ray as part of my daily hospital rounds. I obtained the newest x-ray and compared it with the previous films. That day I saw a new mass that had appeared at the site of Kevin's chest surgery.

When I put the series of films together I thought that a film taken two weeks earlier might have shown the beginning of the mass. I took the films to a staff radiologist and asked for her opinion.

"Yes, you're right. There is something growing near the site of the previous surgery. It's probably a recurrence."

Her words confirmed what I had already concluded. In a period of less than six months, Kevin's lung cancer had indeed recurred.

I hesitated to tell Kevin the news—he had been so elated with the report of the brain studies that did not reveal malignancy. I decided to call Dr. Martini first. We agreed that Kevin should have repeated breathing tests and a chest CAT scan and be seen at Memorial the next week.

I wanted to have this plan in place so that I could tell my patient that a course of action was already set. By this time in our relationship Kevin could read my face so well that when I entered his hospital room, he asked immediately, "What's wrong?"

I told him of the x-ray findings and that he would see Dr. Martini next week for consideration of another operation.

"I feel like a ping-pong ball, back and forth," he moaned. "How can this keep happening? One moment I'm cancer free and the next I'm terminal?" He looked at me, his eyes demanding a comment.

"I think the mass can be removed even though you might have to lose your right lung. You won't be running the marathon but you *will* be able to do most routine things." Kevin paused for a moment, and then said, "As long as I'm alive, I don't care. Let's get on with it."

It was the first time I saw doubt in his expression. He must be wondering whether he could survive much longer. I wasn't sure myself. There was a long silence between us; then he added bleakly, "My girlfriend's left me. She's probably doing the smart thing," he added philosophically. He followed that piece of unhappy news with a touch of his old spirit.

"Hey, Frank, can I get a pass to leave the hospital? I just want to get away for a few hours before I go into surgery again."

While recuperating from brain surgery and finishing the radiation treatments, Kevin was housed in a part of the hospital designed for ambulatory patients not needing much nursing care. The facility resembles a hotel more than a hospital and I knew that from time to time patients go out of the hospital for walks.

"The hospital can't give out passes because they're liable for what happens to you outside of the facility, but I do know that many patients leave for short walks."

Kevin flashed his old mischievous grin.

"Okay then. What they don't know won't hurt them."

The next morning the nurse assigned to Kevin greeted me.

"Your patient had quite a night. He was singing at the top of his lungs when he got back from his 'walk' and you could smell alcohol from the other side of his room. I know what he's going through so I got him into bed and didn't report it."

Kevin had made yet another understanding friend and I thanked her. When I got to Kevin's room on my morning rounds I found him with the shades drawn, blocking out the light.

"Not so loud," he protested as I began to speak in my normal voice. "God, what a hangover!" he whispered.

I reminded him gently that he shouldn't drink alcohol while on powerful medications. He gave a sheepish smirk.

"I know, but I had to get something out of my system. I might not live much longer and Dr. Martini is sharpening up his scalpel, so I just let loose."

But Kevin had had more than just alcohol. He took me by surprise with his next query.

"I know you're a lung specialist, but can you treat venereal disease?"

After requesting the appropriate tests I entered an order for Kevin to receive penicillin. The same nurse, who looked the other way the night before, saw the order and winked.

"I guess this penicillin must be for his bronchitis, Doctor."

I nodded with a straight face, "Yes, but I don't think he will need anymore penicillin after today."

The following day Kevin was seen by Dr. Martini and entered Memorial for his third chest surgery. His right chest was opened through the same incision that had been made five months earlier. Dr. Martini encountered many adhesions from the previous surgery but after careful dissection he was able to free the remaining middle and upper lobes of the right lung. A large tumor mass was found forming in the middle lobe, extending into the upper division. Dr. Martini knew that he would have to remove Kevin's entire right lung in order to completely resect his tumor. Kevin's oxygen level had dropped several times while he was just dissecting the adhesions around the right lung. If he proceeded with the resection, Kevin's remaining left lung might not be able to support his breathing.

At this point, Dr. Martini decided not to remove the right middle and upper lobes. A radiation oncologist was called into the operating room and Dr. Martini described the problem to him.

The radiation oncologist suggested the implantation of radioactive seeds. The radioactive pellets give off a large amount radiation directly into the tumor, killing cancer cells. This large amount of radiation cannot be given in the conventional external method. Although this radioactive seeding had not been used frequently for lung cancer, a few patients prior to Kevin had been treated at Memorial with this technique and the majority had benefited.

The two doctors concluded that Kevin should be treated with radioactive pellets or seeds, placed at the site of the recurrent cancer. Approximately 130 seeds were implanted and Dr. Martini closed his patient's chest.

In addition to the internal radiation of the seeds, Kevin was also given conventional external radiation treatments over a period of four weeks. Kevin phoned me frequently from Memorial. He had not lost his sense of humor.

"I'm glowing in the dark, and they told me to avoid pregnant women since I'll be giving off radiation for the next few months. If your furnace goes on the fritz, I'm available at a small charge."

I asked him if he was disappointed that he had not had the larger surgery and I heard some of his old confidence.

"No way. They tell me the seeds may buy me a few years. At least I'll be able to breathe well while I'm still around."

Kevin's seeds bought him more than a few years. His lung cancer never recurred. Both Dr. Martini and I followed Kevin closely for the five years following his last chest surgery; there was no evidence of recurrence. We became more and more encouraged. Kevin's treatment, however, did not come without a price. In the six months after receiving the huge amount of radiation he began to resemble an atomic blast victim. The main radiation toxicity hit his digestive tract and Kevin lost 50 pounds over a period of a few months because he had difficulty eating and often vomited.

I referred him to a gastroenterologist who performed an examination called endoscopy. In this procedure, a fiberoptic scope is placed into the throat, down the feeding tube called the esophagus and into the stomach. Kevin's esophagus was found to be wider than normal and it did not show the normal muscle tone required to propel food into the stomach. Multiple ulcers were found in the lower esophagus from the reflux of gastric acid. The gastroenterologist concluded that the large amount of radiation had permanently damaged Kevin's esophagus and placed him on medications to reduce acid and improve motility. Gradually Kevin regained lost pounds and after two years he was near his pre-operative weight. He still had to eat very carefully to avoid excessive acid and regurgitation.

A cure from lung cancer is defined by living cancer-free for five years. Five years to the day of the radioactive seeds implantation, I received a call from Dr. Martini who reminded me of Kevin's "anniversary."

"I have your smiling patient here and he's on his way to see you too. He's walking on air." Kevin arrived in my office an hour later with a bottle of champagne.

"I know you can't drink this now but I want to take you and Laurie out to dinner tonight. I have some big news."

We met Kevin later that evening and he announced that he was leaving the area and moving to Florida.

"My parents are there and I'm not finding the type of work I want here. I'll be coming back at least once a year to see you and I'll phone you a lot between visits."

Over the next ten years Kevin returned once a year as promised showing no recurrence of his cancer. On one visit he said proudly, "You won't believe what I'm doing now. I'm working for a cancer society, counseling patients! I take calls on a hot line and give advice. My main message is what you taught me, 'don't give up, always get another opinion, and keep fighting.'"

He handed me a local Florida newspaper feature about him and his new career. In the article he referred to me as the "architect of my great escape from cancer." I thanked him, telling him how pleased I was about this newly found sense of purpose, but reminded him that the fierce desire to survive had come from within him, not me.

After he left, I thought gratefully of how he must be inspiring callers with the amazing story of how he had beaten lung cancer with three chest surgeries, two brain surgeries, and intense radiation treatments.

But there is still another chapter to his story.

On Kevin's visit the following year he reported a disturbing new symptom.

"I'm having trouble with my vision. Certain things I just can't see."

Although the examination I gave him and the review of a new x-ray showed no changes, I advised him, "This may be nothing, or it may be something like cataracts, but I think you should see an ophthalmologist as soon as possible."

Kevin did what I suggested when he returned to Florida. I received a call from him the following week.

"There *is* something wrong. The eye doctor found that I'm not seeing objects off to my left side. He asked me to see a neurologist and to have an MRI."

I encouraged him to follow these recommendations and wondered if it was possible that these findings were due to his previous cancer treatments.

A week later I received a call from a neurosurgeon in Florida asking for information on Kevin's medical history. He said that Kevin's MRI had shown a mass on the outside of the right side of Kevin's brain which was pressing on the right occipital lobe. This put pressure on the nerves that control vision and producing vision problems.

I told him Kevin's history and he said, "I have to see his records but from what you are describing this mass is right near his previous surgery. I think it's a benign tumor, a meningioma. Certainly 15 years after his lung cancer, it cannot be a recurrence. I plan to operate tomorrow and will call you as soon as I get the pathologist's report."

Meningiomas are benign growths that arise from the outer covering of the brain, which is called the meninges. They cause symptoms by growing and pressing on the surrounding brain tissue. Though it did not seem possible that Kevin's lung cancer could have recurred so many years later it was disturbing to hear the new tumor was located almost exactly where he had had his craniotomy and brain radiation. My fears were confirmed the next day.

The neurosurgeon found a malignant tumor had invaded Kevin's brain and he was unable to remove it. The pathology report showed a *sarcoma*, a rare cancer arising from the soft tissues of the body and may occur in many different locations. I called the radiation oncologist who had treated Kevin and asked him what he thought of these findings.

"My God, that's very rare. It's called 'radiation-induced sarcoma.' The reason it's so rare is that most patients don't live long enough after their treatment to develop it. It usually occurs 10 to 15 years post treatment. It's almost as if your patient lived too long."

I didn't agree. I turned to my library of journal articles and found to my regret that the prognosis for a "radiation-induced sarcoma" was very poor. I spoke to Kevin a few days later, who still spoke firmly.

"I heard the news from an oncologist. They want to start me on chemo. Can you check it out?"

I called Kevin's Florida physician and conferred with an oncologist that I worked with. I then called Kevin.

We discussed whether he should return to New York for treatment, but I told him, "The drugs they want to give you in Florida are just what you would receive if you were here in New York."

"What do you think of the chemo treatment they're talking about?"

"It's your best chance."

"As long as the treatment is the same, I'll stay here and keep you posted. I'd like to be near my parents. Guess this is déjà vu all over again."

Still the same old Kevin, still with a sense of humor.

Kevin received one cycle of chemotherapy but about a month later I received a call from his mother.

"Kevin's back in the hospital. He had a seizure and he's not doing well." Her voice broke, but she gave me his phone number and I reached him a few minutes later. I knew from his voice that pain medication was making him groggy, since his speech was slightly slurred.

"The seizure drugs make me dopey and they tell me that the cancer is spreading," he managed to get out.

I rang the oncologist and asked her for more information.

"The new MRI shows the mass is growing. Something has spread to his chest, too. I plan to change his chemotherapy but it doesn't look good."

I called Kevin back and repeated what the oncologist had told me. It was our last conversation. This time his words were clear and he remained defiant.

"I've decided to come to New York and let you take over. Do what you did before, get the best people. I want to give it my best shot."

I promised to do my best and would arrange consultations with both a neurosurgeon and an oncologist. He seemed heartened by my response and said, "Just find me another Dr. Martini."

I made appointments for Kevin for the following week, but on the day he was to arrive his mother phoned.

"Kevin went into a coma the day after you spoke to him. He died last night. I want you to know that his spirits really lifted after your conversation. He seemed to relax and he died peacefully. I know he would want me to thank you for all you've done for him all these years. And I thank you too."

We spoke for several minutes about Kevin and how he and I were more than doctor and patient. My eyes are damp even now, these many years later, as I think of him.

I have told Kevin's story of survival to many cancer patients, and about how I admired his positive, defiant attitude, fighting back against illness. Numerous studies and many other doctors have documented increased lengths of survival in cancer patients who possess the positive attitude that Kevin had.

Did Kevin live too long? I have no doubt about what his answer to that question would be, even with all the pain he went through.

"I have not lived enough."

5

Questions and Answers

o o o o o o o o o o o o o o o o o o o o o o o o o o o o o o o o o o o o o

The Important Thing is Not to Stop Questioning

—Einstein

Shortness of breath is one of the most common problems a lung specialist encounters, its medical term being *dyspnea*, from the Greek word meaning *bad breathing*. I often refer to this disturbing symptom as "air hunger" and many patients describe the sensation as "not being able to get enough air."

For the physician, determining the source of dyspnea can be extremely challenging because there are so many possibilities, including anxiety. A careful, step-by-step approach is needed to arrive at the correct diagnosis. Once the source of dyspnea is identified, a specific treatment may follow, allowing the patient to return to normal breathing and a full and active life. This process of discovery and correction, if successful can be extremely rewarding—not only for the patient but the doctor as well.

This was so in the case for my patient, Joseph Marino, who was referred to me by another patient, a physician whom I had treated successfully for pneumonia.

The first day he came to see me, Joseph sat motionless in my consultation room, his breathing rapid and labored; he was in obvious distress. His son Joe Jr. had accompanied him, and he sat with us as I began my customary questioning.

"Can you describe the problem that brought you here today?"

It was a moment or so before he could speak. "I can't breathe," he gasped.

It was difficult for him to say even those three words. His son began to offer details of his father's medical history in order to save his father the effort of speaking.

I learned that Joseph had no prior problem with breathing. Sixty-nine years old, holding both business and law degrees, he was the CEO of a large company and was accustomed to giving speeches, holding daily staff meetings and organizing conferences. I could tell quickly that he was used to being the boss.

"I need to get back to work soon and I hear you're the man to get me well," he managed to say for himself without his son's help. The unspoken words were, "and do it fast!"

Joseph's past medical history was unremarkable except for a small stroke two years before his current illness. I made a note that he had formerly smoked two packs of cigarettes a day but had stopped almost 30 years ago. Joe Jr. related that his father worked long hours and exercised frequently up until three weeks prior to this meeting

"No one can keep up with him either at work or on the tennis court."

A medical history can often be straightforward and routine, but Joseph's was about to turn into a good mystery novel, and I was going to have to be the chief detective.

His son began the story: Just five days before seeing me, Joseph had been discharged from a local hospital where he was hospitalized for three weeks because of the sudden onset of pain in his right buttock that radiated down his right leg.

This type of pain is often called *sciatica* since it reflects pressure on the sciatic nerve that exits the spinal cord in the low back or lumbar area and branches to supply nerve impulses to both legs. Joseph had had less severe but similar pain before and a back problem for many years. On admission to the hospital a staff neurologist prescribed bed rest with morphine for pain and ordered an MRI of his spine. The MRI was done the next day. It confirmed a suspected herniated disc in the lumbar region, which was treated with bed rest and pain medication. A spinal disc is made up of a gelatinous material that acts as a cushion between two spinal bones called vertebrae. When this material slips out of its normal position, it presses down on nerve fibers that make up the sciatic nerve, creating pain.

On the seventh day of his hospitalization Joseph awoke with nausea, restlessness, and severe shortness of breath.

"I didn't know what was happening. I just couldn't breathe."

He called for his nurse, who found him lethargic and breathing rapidly. An intern drew blood from an artery in his wrist for a blood gas analysis. The result was striking, revealing a lowered oxygen level of 59 (normal is above 80) as well as a low level of carbon dioxide of 26 (normal is 40). Joseph's rapid breathing had lowered his carbon dioxide level but his oxygen level remained low. The admitting neurologist thought he might have suffered another stroke or developed a pulmonary embolus and so ordered an MRI of the brain as well as a chest x-ray and lung scan.

A pulmonary embolus is a blood clot that originates in a blood vessel in another part of the body, usually the legs or pelvis, and travels through the circulation to lodge in a blood vessel in the lung. Once in the lung the clot usually fragments, sending smaller pieces into smaller blood vessels. This condition is one of the most common complications of bed rest or immobilization so I understood why Joseph's physicians considered it.

The diagnosis of a pulmonary embolus is often made by a lung scan in which a radioactive tracer is injected into a vein and also inhaled. A scanner that detects radioactivity can then track where the tracer goes. If a clot has lodged in a blood vessel the scan will show a defect in that area of the lung. Unfortunately a lung scan may be abnormal from other chest problems, making the diagnosis of a pulmonary embolus difficult. Joseph's lung scan was read by the radiologist as "indeterminate" since a single defect was seen in the lower right lung where his chest x-ray showed atelectasis. His physicians then ordered a pulmonary angiogram. In this more invasive test, a thin catheter is inserted into a large vein in the groin and passed through the circulation and heart until it is positioned in the arteries leading to the lungs. Once in position, the radiologist injects dye to outline the blood vessels. If a clot has lodged in these vessels, filling defects, which are empty areas where blood cannot go due to the presence of clots, are visualized and the diagnosis of embolism is confirmed.

Both Joseph's brain MRI and pulmonary angiogram proved normal. A few hours after these tests, he felt better and a repeat test of his oxygen level showed 75. He had received no treatment so his physicians were puzzled by his sudden, spontaneous recovery. Joseph's improvement, however, was short-lived.

The next day he again developed severe shortness of breath and rapid breathing. A repeat blood gas test now showed an oxygen level of 50. Consultations were set up with cardiology and pulmonary physicians. Once again Joseph improved spontaneously only to develop a third and fourth similar episode over the next several days. His back pain also lessened and he began to walk, experiencing shortness of breath while taking just a few steps.

"I knew something was still very wrong. I really wasn't well even between the attacks."

The consulting heart specialist reviewed Joseph's heart tracing or electrocardiogram (EKG). The possibility of a heart attack had to be considered because of his history of having had a stroke. The EKG did not reveal heart damage and an echocardiogram or "echo" was taken. An echocardiogram uses high-frequency sound waves to examine the heart. In a routine study, a technician or sonographer applies a conductive jelly to the patient's chest and then applies a wand called a transducer that emits and then receives the reflected sound waves. These reflections produce a detailed image, like radar or sonar that can be viewed and recorded. Echocardiograms may also use a device called *Doppler* that measures blood movement or flow. The sounds of blood flow through the heart may then also be heard and recorded. Joseph's echocardiogram proved normal.

The consulting lung specialist obtained breathing tests called "Pulmonary Function Tests," which measure the capacity of the lungs and the distribution of air within them, as well as showing how air flows in and out of the bronchial tubes and the exchange within the small air sacs or alveoli. Joseph's results were again normal. At this point a technician applied a tight face mask in order to deliver a high concentration of oxygen. A blood gas was obtained before and after this application. Room air consists of

21% oxygen; the air mixture given to Joseph consisted of 100% oxygen. This is commonly referred to as a "test for shunting."

The human heart is divided into right and left halves by a thick muscular wall called the septum. Each half of the heart is divided into an upper and lower chamber. The upper, smaller chambers are called the *atria* and the lower, larger chambers are called the *ventricles*. A door-like valve allows blood to enter and leave each chamber. In the normal circulation the left side of the heart pumps oxygen-enriched blood that it has received from the lungs to the various body organs. This oxygenated blood travels through vessels called arteries so that it is called arterial. Once the organs take up oxygen, the oxygen depleted blood travels back through vessels called veins to the right side of the heart and then into the lungs. In the lungs, this venous blood is distributed to the air sacs in tiny vessels called capillaries where oxygen is re-supplied and carbon dioxide excreted. These vessels then merge into larger channels that return the oxygen enriched blood to the left side of the heart and the cycle begins again.

When 100% oxygen is breathed, the level of oxygen in the air sacs of the lung rises to a very high level. Oxygen then transfers to the blood in the adjacent pulmonary capillaries. A sample of arterial blood should then reveal a very high oxygen level. Joseph breathed the high oxygen mixture for twenty minutes and then a blood gas sample was taken. The result was perplexing. His oxygen level had only risen from 59 to 65! As I obtained this information from Joseph and his medical records, I knew instantly that this relatively simple test held the answer to Joseph's problem.

A portion of his venous blood was not being enriched with the inhaled oxygen. The reduced level of oxygen was then detected by nerve receptors that relayed this distress signal to the brain, producing the sensation of shortness of breath. Joseph had what is called medically a "shunt," a site in the body where blood could bypass the air sacs and capillaries of the lungs.

Where was it located? Blood was being transferred from one side of his circulation to the other without going through the capillaries of the lung. Joseph's physicians at the other hospital and I knew that the two most common shunts are blood vessel connections called A-V malformations and defects within the heart. Joseph's lung x-rays and scans did not show such a lung malformation and his echocardiogram had been read as normal. If a shunt existed, why did it seemingly open and close, allowing Joseph to improve without any treatment? The physicians at the other hospital termed Joseph's case "baffling" and suggested he be seen at a referral center.

After hearing this suggestion I examined Joseph again myself and found his lungs clear. I listened carefully to his heart but heard only normal heart sounds. I repeated his breathing tests and oxygen measurements and found very similar results to those recorded at the other hospital. While doing the exam and waiting for the completion of the testing, I considered what the next steps should be. I then sat down with Joseph and Joe Jr. and explained what a shunt meant and my plan of action.

"I believe you do have a shunt. It just hasn't been detected yet. With so many clear chest x-rays, we can exclude a malformation in your lungs. That leaves only your heart as the suspect location."

Joseph interrupted, "But my echo was normal. How could it be my heart?"

I was about to tell him how we could find out. It would be an innovative approach to the problem.

During the same period that I was seeing Joseph, a new echo technique had just been put into use called transesophageal echocardiography or TEE. In this technique the transducer that emits the sound waves is attached to a fiberoptic scope, which is swallowed by the patient and comes to rest in the digestive passage called the esophagus. The esophagus is a hollow tube that begins in the back of the throat and travels down through the chest to empty into the stomach. By emitting sound waves from within the chest rather than from the surface of the skin as in a regular echocardiogram, the TEE technique provides a more detailed image of the heart and its chambers.

I explained to Joseph that his regular echo might just have missed the shunt and that the TEE would create a better image.

"I think this might give us the answer," I reassured him.

He instantly agreed to being admitted to the hospital for this test, saying, "Let's get it done."

Joseph underwent the TEE study the next morning. First his throat was numbed with a Novocain-like anesthetic spray and then he swallowed the long fiberoptic scope to the desired depth to position it within the center of his chest near his heart.

In the thirty-plus years since I graduated from medical school, some of the technological advances in medicine of today never cease to astound me. Although many years have passed I still remember sitting down with my hospital's echocardiographer to go over the tape recording of Joseph's echo. I had seen routine echocardiograms many times but this was my first TEE. I believe one of the reasons I can still picture the results is that so many of my senses were stimulated by this study. I was used to seeing echos in black and white so I was struck by the bright, dynamic color images of Joseph's heart. One color represented the muscle tissue of the heart while another flashed with the flow of blood. The study also incorporated the Doppler technique so that the pulsing, whooshing sounds of blood flowing through the valves and chambers of the heart reverberated around the small, darkened room. Perhaps the anticipation of learning the answer to Joseph's medical mystery also heightened my appreciation of the laser-like display of information. Joseph's son sat in with us and his awed expression mirrored my own amazement.

The echocardiographer began to describe the dancing images before us and I could tell from his voice that although he had seen thousands of echos, he was also excited by the findings and this new technique. He brought the tape to a point where the image clearly showed the four chambers of the heart. Pointing to the level of the atria he said, "Now watch this."

I saw a streak of color pass from the right side of the heart to the left. After a few seconds, it was clear that with each pulsation of Joseph's heart, a jet of blood was passing from right to left.

"That's an atrial septal defect (ASD), and now I'm going to show you more proof. The technician has just injected into your patient's vein a saline contrast solution. This solution contains harmless microscopic bubbles. If the diagnosis of an ASD is correct the bubbles will show up in seconds on the left side of the heart."

Pointing to the screen he said, "Keep your eyes here." Just as he predicted, little tiny round bubble defects suddenly appeared within the color swatch of the left side of Joseph's heart. The saline had traveled through a vein into the right side of the heart and then passed through an opening in the wall between the two atria, completely bypassing the lungs and the oxygen containing alveoli. With obvious pride, he pronounced, "There is no doubt. You have your diagnosis. It's an ASD."

An atrial septal defect is an opening between the two upper chambers of the heart. It is the most common type of congenital heart disease in adolescents and adults. ASDs vary in size from a few millimeters to several centimeters. Some atrial defects present at birth may close spontaneously by the age of five. Depending on the size of the defect, an ASD may remain undiscovered for life, especially with a tiny opening. At birth the pressures on the two sides of the heart are nearly equal but the pressures in the right chambers quickly decrease so that the direction of flow of blood in most ASDs is from left to right. When blood flows from the left side of the heart to the right, blood oxygen levels do not fall since oxygen may be picked up within the lungs with each pass through. Over time, however, the right-sided chambers of the heart enlarge from the extra flow of blood from the left and become stiffer, eventually reversing the direction of blood flow. This had clearly occurred in Joseph's case while he was hospitalized for his slipped disc.

But what accounted for Joseph's "attacks" when his oxygen level plummeted, only to mysteriously increase? The answer was also found during the TEE study. One of the maneuvers that the sonographer performed during the TEE is called a Valsalva. The patient is asked to bear down as if to have a bowel movement. This effort results in an increase of blood flow back to the heart from the extremities and internal organs. As the returning blood filled the right side of Joseph's heart, an increased amount passed from right to left, causing a sudden drop in his oxygen level. Other changes in Joseph's activity and position might have also increased the flow of blood from right to left producing the attacks.

Joseph's mysterious improvement was likely due to periods of relaxation of the heart muscle when less blood filled the right-sided chambers of the heart and the right to left flow through the ASD was reduced. Joseph's "baffling case" had been solved. I knew that if his ASD could be successfully closed he would return to a full and active life.

One of the true miracles of modern medicine is the ability to operate on the human heart. Dr. John Gibbon developed the heart-lung machine in 1953. This device acts as an artificial heart during the time that the heart must be stopped so that the surgeon can work on an immobile organ. The heart-lung machine receives the patient's blood, removes carbon dioxide, adds oxygen, and pumps the blood back through the body. This machine, however, may cause small clots to form in the blood that passes through, which can cause stroke or kidney failure. To avoid this problem, a new technique called "minimally invasive cardiac surgery" has been developed. In this procedure, surgeons make a small incision in the chest and operate while the heart continues to beat.

However, at the time of Joseph's hospitalization, the "minimally invasive" technique was still considered experimental. Joseph's cardiac surgeon considered both approaches but decided to proceed with traditional surgery.

True to the impatient personality I recognized from the moment I met him, Joseph wanted the surgery to be done as soon as possible. A team of physicians—a cardiologist, an anesthesiologist and a cardiac surgeon—was quickly assembled with the patient's approval and the surgery was scheduled. I visited Joseph the night before and told him that my role would be to monitor his lung function in the post-operative period. He thanked me for putting together the team of physicians that would repair his heart.

I asked if he was nervous and he said, "I figure I have gotten the best advice and have the best surgeon, so I'm just thinking of how much better my tennis game will be." I promised to see him in the recovery room after the surgery.

Early the next morning the cardiac surgeon first made a foot-long incision through the center of Joseph's breastbone or sternum. After being attached to the heart-lung machine, Joseph's heart was stopped with the application of a cold solution containing potassium. The right atrium was opened revealing a large atrial septal defect measuring 1.5 centimeters in diameter. The surgeon then closed the defect with sutures. The heart was restarted with an electric shock and the patient was removed from the heart-lung machine. Blood gases were taken which showed Joseph's oxygen level close to normal.

I saw Joseph that evening and found him sedated, breathing with the help of a respirator, and noted that the reading of his oxygen level on a nearby monitor was normal and that he was receiving only a low level of oxygen. Within twelve hours, Joseph was breathing on his own, though with an oxygen mask. Within a few days he was breathing freely, without distress and no supportive oxygen.

When I visited the last time before his discharge, I found him packing his bag by himself and he was having no trouble speaking or moving about. He greeted me with a smile, and said, "It's amazing. I'm no longer short of breath. I can really breathe again."

Joseph quickly returned to work and the tennis court. I still occasionally receive updates from his cardiac surgeon and hear he is doing exceptionally well. His case is a true success story, one of the many miracles of modern medicine.

In my practice I find that each day is a mix of uplifting cases like Joseph's and less successful outcomes. After many years in medicine, the cases that end well have become ever more satisfying, while those that do not, I have come to accept, though reluctantly.

Surgeons now frequently repair heart problems with the patient's heart still beating, avoiding the risks of the heart-lung machine. The TEE study is now considered routine for the diagnosis of many cardiac illnesses. Patients are often admitted and discharged after cardiac surgery within a few days. Medicine and technology advance daily to provide more accurate diagnoses and better treatments. Complications of surgery and treatment failures, however, also persist, so that a physician can never be satisfied with the status quo.

When I see young doctors today ordering a TEE or preparing a patient for cardiac surgery, I stop to wonder, do they see medical advances and techniques with the thrill I do, never taking breakthroughs for granted.

My hope is that they also will be forever astounded by the miracle of the human body and know the inner fulfillment that comes with solving a medical mystery.

6

Polio Revisited

Courage is the thing. All goes if courage goes.

—*J.M. Barrie*

Everyone in the hospital was eager to see the man with the carbon dioxide (CO_2) level of 97, a near-death level of what is potentially a poison gas. Residents, interns, and medical students were waiting for him to arrive in the Intensive Care Unit.

I had just come up to the ICU from the emergency room to brief the house officers about the patient in question. Word of his impending arrival and abnormal blood gases had preceded me. I was met with a round of questions.

"Is he comatose?" "Did he arrest?" "Is he intubated?"

Seventy-one-year-old Seth Howard was admitted to the hospital through the emergency room with complaints of dizziness and shortness of breath. His attending physician, a cardiologist who had treated him for heart disease for several years, asked me to see him. My role as a pulmonologist was to evaluate this gentleman's breathing while a neurologist was called to evaluate the dizziness.

I found Seth in the emergency room on a stretcher, surrounded by nurses and ER physicians. He was a thin, pale man who seemed very composed despite all the flurry and hubbub around him. After introducing myself, I began the process of obtaining a medical history.

With any new patient, a physician attempts to elicit a detailed, factual accounting of the present and past medical history. While interviewing, I also observe the patient for signs or clues to his disease. His chief complaint was that he was dizzy and that he had difficulty walking as a result.

"I lose my balance and I'm constantly short of breath. It's gotten worse the last few weeks. I just can't seem to get enough air."

He told of having to take frequent stops to catch his breath while walking, and of waking up at night unable to breathe.

"I have to open the window to try to get some air. Doesn't help much."

After hearing about the recent events, I turned to Seth's past medical history.

"Did you have any lung problems as a child?"

"I had polio when I was twelve, and it produced paralysis of my arms and legs. I recovered slowly but was left with permanent muscle weakness."

I could see that those weakened muscles of his back and torso had also produced a deformity of his spine, known as scoliosis. This condition is a pronounced curvature of the spine, which often distorts the chest cavity, producing a restriction in the expansion of the lungs. Seth had had several operations on his spine as a child but had been left with a severe curve. Despite these major problems that affected his everyday movements, he had worked hard to lead a normal life, and he had run a successful business. He was married and had two children.

Seth was an intelligent, pleasant man who asked the right questions such as "How do you get the carbon dioxide down?" but volunteered little information. He reminded me of the Joe Friday character, offering "just the facts" and little else. He spoke as if his childhood polio, multiple surgeries, years of rehabilitation had been routine; he minimized the pain and disability that I knew he must have experienced.

Some medical histories are taken with the difficulty of a tooth extraction and this was a good example of such an interview. I had to inquire several times to get any details of his childhood experiences with physicians and therapists.

"I was lucky," he said. "My best friend got polio just before I did. He had to live in an iron lung. He never came home."

While listening to a medical history I try to assess the patient's inner drive and strength, looking for an insight into the patient's character. I knew that Seth must have a strong life force, having gone through all that he had in the past, but I had difficulty seeing beyond his exterior stoicism. I decided to focus on my patient's immediate problem but planned to continue questioning him about his previous history after his condition stabilized.

During the interview Seth's breathing rate was faster than normal and his lips and fingernails had a bluish hue. This is called *cyanosis*, produced when blood oxygen levels are low. I reviewed his blood tests and noted that Seth's level of bicarbonate was high. Very high.

The lung functions to obtain oxygen (O_2), which is the fuel for body functions, and to excrete a waste product—carbon dioxide (CO_2). When an illness reduces the expansion of the lungs, the reduced capacity may result in increased CO_2 levels. As CO_2 rises, oxygen levels fall, resulting in cyanosis. When CO_2 increases, there is also a shift in the chemical balance of the body towards a more acidic environment called *acidosis*. If this happens rapidly, it may prove fatal. A gradual increase in CO_2, however, can be balanced by a compensatory mechanism in which the levels of a base substance called bicarbonate increases. This adjustment brings the chemical balance of the body back towards normal.

Another abnormality in Seth's blood indicating an imbalance in the exchange of oxygen was an elevated red blood cell count. The red blood cells carry oxygen throughout the body to act as the fuel for body functions. Oxygen is bound to a substance known as *hemoglobin*, contained within the red blood cells. When there is a lack of oxygen, the body attempts to compensate by producing a larger number of these cells. The increase in the amount of oxygen delivered to various organs by this mechanism, however, is not very great and may produce a serious adverse effect. If the increase in the number of red blood cells is marked, they may actually clog small blood vessels reducing the flow of blood to vital organs.

One of the tools a pulmonologist uses in evaluating a patient with a breathing disorder is a blood gas test, directly measuring the levels of oxygen and CO_2 in the blood. I sampled Seth's blood from an artery in his wrist. The normal level of CO_2 is 40 millimeters of mercury (mmHg). The normal level of O_2 is 80 mmHg. Seth's blood gas revealed a CO_2 of 97 and an O_2 of 29 as well as acidosis. I decided to repeat the sampling to be sure there had been no error. The repeat sample revealed a CO_2 of 102. His condition was deteriorating.

For Seth to be alert and speaking, it was clear that his body had adjusted to these striking changes in his blood gases. This adjustment may occur when the elevation in CO_2 is very gradual, allowing compensation for the acidosis. Many patients are also able to adapt to low oxygen levels, demonstrated by the populations of the world who live at high altitudes and suffer no lasting adverse effects.

Nevertheless, the hospital house officers expected to receive a comatose patient because when these changes in blood gases occur suddenly, the patient loses consciousness and expires unless he can be resuscitated. Although Seth's compensatory mechanisms had allowed him to survive, the low oxygen level had by now produced shortness of breath and a more rapid breathing rate.

Normal breathing is effortless. When breathing rates increase, however, increased energy is needed as fuel for the muscles that cause the lungs to expand. Doctors call this energy expenditure the "work of breathing." Like all muscles, those that are used to inflate the lungs may tire. When fatigue strikes the breathing muscles, lung expansion decreases causing decreased air movement and a further elevation of CO_2.

A low oxygen level is always dangerous because it is the fuel that maintains normal body function. Some body tissues are extremely sensitive to a lack of oxygen. The heart is one example. When oxygen levels fall in the heart, the muscle may be damaged, producing a heart attack that can weaken its action. This may result in heart failure or an irregular heart beat. Seth had endured heart disease for several years so that the added insult of a low oxygen level made his situation even more serious.

It was clear from Seth's history and the analysis of his blood that he was experiencing failure of the respiratory system that sustains life. Without treatment the low oxygen would eventually produce damage to his heart or brain. As the acidosis progressed further, a life threatening irregular heart rhythm might "arrest" or stop his heart.

Why had this happened? What had produced this catastrophic derangement in the inner environment of his body?

The answer was in his medical history.

Poliomyelitis is a viral infection that attacks the nervous system, disabling muscles and sometimes suffocating its victims. The first recorded epidemic of polio in the United States occurred in Vermont in 1894. In 1916, 6,000 people died from the virus and 27,000 were paralyzed. In New York City during the week of August 5, 1916 there were 1,151 reported cases of polio with 301 deaths. This outbreak caused widespread panic, with police breaking into homes to take suspected polio virus carriers into custody. Cats and dogs were impounded because they were mistakenly thought to carry the virus.

Between 1940 and 1944 there were an estimated 10,000 cases a year in the United States. Between 1945 and 1949, the average jumped to 24,000 a year. Outbreaks always occurred during the summer months, the worst outbreaks coming every three years. Swimming pools were closed and summer camps for children went out of business.

In the most common type of polio, called spinal poliomyelitis, the virus attacks the nerve cells that control the muscles of the limbs, trunk, diaphragm, abdomen, and pelvis. In bulbar poliomyelitis, the most deadly form of the disease, the nerve cells of the brain stem are affected. This vital area of the central nervous system controls swallowing, eye movements, and breathing. Patients with bulbar polio usually required an "iron lung" to breathe.

The polio virus attacks nerve cells called motor neurons that control muscle function, producing paralysis and weakness. In an average case of paralytic poliomyelitis, 95% of motor neurons are infected, and 50% of those neurons die. Depending on the number of neurons involved, the result ranges from muscle weakness to complete paralysis. Many polio survivors remember having muscles that were completely paralyzed begin to move again after a period of a few weeks. The greatest return of muscle function occurs within the first six months, but improvement may continue for up to two years. Over this time period, many polio survivors regained strength and mobility and were able to discard braces or wheelchairs.

The increasing numbers of polio cases in the 1940s prompted a vigorous research effort that focused on the development of a vaccine. It had been shown that once a person was infected with the polio virus, antibodies against the virus were manufactured, creating immunity. A trial of a polio vaccine was initiated in 1954 in 44 states. On April 12, 1955, Dr. Thomas Francis, Jr., a University of Michigan scientist, and Dr. Jonas Salk of the University of Pittsburgh, reported that Salk's polio vaccine was safe, effective and potent. Science had triumphed over the crippling disease.

But the story was not over. Beginning in the 1970s and 1980s, polio survivors began reporting a cluster of symptoms now referred to as "*post polio syndrome,*" or PPS. The number of survivors of paralytic polio in this country is estimated to be 1.63 million. Approximately 25 to 40% of these individuals, 40 to 50 years after developing polio, have experienced PPS; it is estimated that 66% to 80% will be affected to some degree.

The characteristic symptoms of PPS are weakness, fatigue, and pain. Shortness of breath, cold intolerance, and difficulty swallowing are also common. The cause of PPS has not been established. Current research favors the theory of chronic disintegration of regenerated nerve cells. These nerve cells were initially injured but not destroyed by the original polio infection. As these cells fatigue or die off, muscles fail to receive stimulation, resulting in weakness. PPS is likely accelerated by the normal aging process, which also reduces the numbers of nerve cells. The average age of patients confronted with PPS is 55; seven was the average age at onset of the original polio infection.

The muscles of the rib cage and the diaphragm—a dome-like muscle that moves up and down with each breath—support breathing. Weakness of these muscles reduces the inflation of the lungs resulting in small lung volumes and impaired exchange of oxygen and carbon dioxide. There is also an increased risk of respiratory infection such as pneumonia because of difficulty in the clearing of secretions.

Seth, a polio victim at age 12, had slowly developed the post-polio syndrome in his seventies, producing respiratory failure.

In addition to shortness of breath, Seth reported he could not cough up mucous to clear his chest. Fortunately, his chest x-ray did not show pneumonia and there were no other signs of infection. His low oxygen and high carbon dioxide levels needed to be treated quickly to prevent organ damage and to reverse the acidotic state.

With each breath, air moves from outside the body through the nose and mouth into the windpipe, bronchial tubes, and air sacs of the lung. This inhalation of air is called inspiration. The movement of air is accomplished by the contraction of breathing muscles. Air moves because of the difference in pressure between the atmosphere and the chest. The pressure within the chest is less than that in the atmosphere. With exhalation or air, or expiration, the pressure gradient reverses, driving air out of the lungs. Expiration is also aided by the elastic nature of the lung, which recoils after expansion.

Seth needed assistance in breathing, an artificial respirator to help him breathe and to allow his fatigued muscles to rest. Ironically, he had not required an "iron lung" when he had developed polio.

Peter Drinker invented the iron lung in 1921. I first encountered this respirator during my fellowship at Bellevue and the Manhattan Veterans Administration Hospitals in 1973. This device was designed to assist breathing by producing a vacuum or negative pressure around the outside of the chest, mimicking the normal action of breathing. In order to achieve this, the patient's chest cavity had to be contained within the chamber. The iron lung resembled a large metal tank or cylinder, lying on its side, opening only at one end where the patient's head was supported by a small platform. An internal "bed," which was really more like a stretcher, slid forward and back, allowing the patient to be placed in and out of the device. Small portals were placed on both sides of the iron lung to allow limited access to the contained patient.

What I remember most about the iron lung is the noise it made. It emitted a hissing and plopping sound as the internal motor cycled, alternating internal negative and positive pressures. Patients were placed in these great metal cylinders for hours at a time, to be removed only for meals or to relieve themselves. At any one time the hospital's intensive care units might have several patients in "tanks" so that patients and staff alike had to adjust to the monotony of these strange sounds.

If technology had not made tremendous strides in the last 50 years, an iron lung would have been necessary to assist Seth in breathing. But thankfully, technology *had* moved forward, initially with smaller negative pressure devices that fit only over the chest itself or body suits that resemble those of a deep-sea diver.

By 1944, the first positive pressure respirator was manufactured. These devices inflate the lung with a set pressure or amount of air. In order to achieve this, the respirator must be connected to the patient by a tube inserted into the windpipe. This insertion is called intubation and is commonly done through the mouth, less frequently via the nose.

Once intubated, the patient is unable to speak, severely reducing the ability to communicate and preventing swallowing. In order to provide nourishment, patients on respirators are usually fed through a feeding tube placed in the stomach. Breathing or endotracheal tubes can only be left in position for relatively short periods because they may produce damage to the voice box. In order to avoid this, patients who require longer periods on a respirator undergo an operation called a tracheotomy in which the breathing tube is transferred to the windpipe, just below the Adam's apple.

Fortunately, technology did not stop with the development of positive pressure respirators. In order to avoid the complications of intubation, devices that assist breathing by providing positive pressure through a face mask have been developed. In some instances, the mask is applied to the nose alone, in others to the entire face, similar to what a jet pilot might wear. Not only do these devices deliver the pressure to inflate the lungs but they also cycle different pressures on inspiration and expiration.

This apparatus is called "Bilevel Positive Airway Pressure" or "BIPAP." It was such a device that I suggested for Seth Howard. This would avoid intubation, allow him to be nourished normally when the mask was off, and communicate with his family and physicians. Would it work?

At the time of Seth's admission to the hospital, BIPAP had been available for only a short time. Although a face mask is more comfortable for the patient than an endotracheal tube, some of the pressure used to expand the lungs is lost, reducing its effectiveness. Just prior to seeing Seth I had seen BIPAP fail in a patient with emphysema and pneumonia who then required intubation.

Seth's problem was different; though PPS had severely weakened his breathing muscles, his lungs were clear. The lower pressures delivered by BIPAP might be adequate to assist his breathing.

Before the application of this device, I explained to Seth and his wife that his breathing was failing and that without respiratory support, he would die. I also had to explain that the new mask device might not work and he would then have to be intubated and attached to a respirator for an indefinite period. I told him that he had the option to decline the respirator, but there would be little chance of survival without it.

Though I have had this type of conversation with patients and their families countless times, it is never easy for me to discuss the consequences of a serious illness and end of life issues. Each patient, each family is unique to me; each time it feels as though it is the first time in my career that I am telling someone they might die.

As I explained the situation fully to Seth and his wife, she wiped away tears. But Seth spoke up firmly.

"It doesn't sound as if I have any other choice. Do what you think is best."

I am not sure if it was the concern on my face or the trappings of a major hospital's intensive care unit, but Seth and his family understood that he was seriously ill.

He continued to demonstrate his "all business" persona. There was no hesitation although his face showed concern and uncertainty.

"When can we get started?"

In many life-threatening situations the rapport between doctor and patient must be established quickly. Seth was willing to trust me although we had met just sixty minutes before. He would tell me later that I had explained his problem in terms he understood.

"You seemed to know what you were talking about—your suggestions made sense to me."

A respiratory therapist brought in the BIPAP with several different sized masks. A tight fit is essential to prevent leakage of air but the mask would have to fit comfortably if Seth were to be able to wear it for hours at a time. Padding at the bridge of the nose was needed to prevent chafing.

The respiratory therapist and I decided on certain pressure settings but these would be adjusted according to Seth's tolerance of the device and blood gas test results. Oxygen was also added to the system. The device was turned on.

After 20 minutes on BIPAP with the initial settings, a blood gas test was repeated. Seth's CO_2 had dropped to 77. He was better but still acidotic. The pressure settings were increased and the amount of O_2 adjusted. Over a period of several hours, his blood gases improved significantly, so that by the next morning, CO_2 levels were near 60 and O_2 levels nearly equal to that. Seth was then allowed to take off the mask and to eat breakfast.

I asked if he had been able to sleep with the face mask and BIPAP during the night.

"Sleep? I don't think I will ever be able to sleep with this thing on. It makes a huge noise and my face feels unbelievably hot."

After several days in the ICU and subsequently in a regular room, the strength in Seth's breathing muscles improved; gradually he was able to be off BIPAP and oxygen during the day and to use the assist device only during the night. His CO_2 level dropped to 55 and his O_2 level breathing room air was 64.

He was discharged from the hospital after two weeks!

Seth had avoided death from polio once again. I had seen him daily while he was hospitalized; frequently I came around several times a day, but never throughout his stay did he ever open up about his past medical experiences.

On a follow-up office visit several months after he was discharged, he said he had conquered his difficulty sleeping with BIPAP and welcomed its use because he felt so much less short of breath in the morning.

I told him how concerned all of us attending physicians had been when he was admitted and how wonderful it was to see him now looking so well.

His expression softened and he said, "You know when I first had polio it was like I grew up overnight. My friends were dying and I was told I might die. What did a kid that age know about illness and death? My childhood ended at twelve."

We spoke for a few minutes then about his past experiences and I saw for the first time beyond his stoic exterior.

"Seth, you showed a great deal of strength and composure during a very stressful illness," I told him sincerely.

He paused for a moment after that. Then he said, "When I was a child, I told myself I couldn't, must never, let fear take over. That vow carried me through then and it carries me through now."

It is now twelve years since Seth Howard was admitted to the hospital and he continues to see me twice a year. He has maintained his use of BIPAP faithfully each night, allowing him to function without support during the day. His muscle weakness still severely limits his activities but his quality of life is good and he has lived to see the birth of two grandchildren.

After twenty-five years in private practice, I am never completely sure why one patient survives and another does not. In Seth's case, I believe he survived not only because of advances in technology but also because of his drive to live and the willingness to trust his life to someone in a white coat whom he had just met. I cherish that trust.

On my daily rounds, I carry the hope that today there will be no new patient to appear in my dreams of lost patients. I am grateful Seth is not among them.

7

Dear Doctor

o o o o o o o o o o o o o o o o o o o o o o o o o o o o o o o o o o

"Hope is the denial of reality."

—*Margaret Weis*

One of my most important tasks as a physician is to educate patients about their illnesses. An informed patient is less likely to suffer an exacerbation of a chronic condition than an individual with little understanding of their ailment.

I spend a good deal of time during office visits just talking with my patients, educating them in layman's terms about their illness. Sometimes we chat about other things of interest to them, laying the groundwork for trust between us.

Unfortunately, my efforts at patient education are not always successful. These failures may occur for a multitude of reasons. In some instances the patient's life experiences have produced an aversion to medication, mistrust of the wisdom of physicians, and/or an unwillingness to accept the fact that they have a chronic illness.

Edith Tannenbaum, an editor of a liberal foreign policy journal who loved politics and the exchange of ideas, was one such person. Discussion of the seriousness of her condition was always something she wanted to avoid on her visits to me.

Edith came to me for treatment of severe asthma. Bronchial asthma is an inflammatory disease of the air passages (bronchial tubes) in which these airways become red, swollen, and irritable. The inflammation and swelling of the internal lining of these tubes as well as constriction of surrounding muscle narrows these passageways. This narrowing produces shortness of breath, coughing and commonly, wheezing. An outpouring of sticky mucus from the inflamed bronchial tubes further closes off air passages, which may become dangerously plugged up.

Asthma is often closely related to allergy but also frequently occurs in non-allergic individuals. Allergic asthmatics usually begin to have symptoms in childhood while the non-allergic patients most usually are adults. Many causes of asthma have been implicated in the non-allergic patients but the majority of cases appear to be triggered by respiratory infections. Death from asthma is rare compared with many other lung diseases—they account for only about 5,000 fatalities a year in this country. These deaths are always tragic because asthma is a treatable, reversible disease in the vast majority of patients.

Allergy is by definition over-sensitivity to substances (*allergens*) that may be inhaled, ingested, or just touched to the skin. In an allergic asthmatic, for example, inhalation of tree pollen may produce a sudden swelling and constriction of the air passages of the lung followed by an acute asthmatic attack. I have always had a special interest in asthma, maybe because I have suffered from hay fever since childhood.

Born in Germany, Edith was a holocaust survivor from Auschwitz who had married another holocaust survivor whom she met on the ship that carried them to the United States. I saw with sadness the tattooed numbers on her forearm during my initial physical examination. Edith spoke with a distinct accent and addressed me as "Dear Doctor," always maintaining a European air of formality with me.

Now 63 years old, Edith told me her husband had died of colon cancer two years before our first visit. They had been unable to have children and she now lived alone in a Manhattan apartment not far from the NYU medical center where I had my office. Edith had developed asthma as an adult long after surviving the concentration camp and immigrating to this country. She was consulting me after landing in the medical center's emergency room because of a severe asthmatic attack.

Adult onset asthma is more difficult to control than the childhood type and Edith was a good example of this generalization. She also had features of a unique form of adult onset asthma associated with three features: longstanding nasal congestion known as *rhinitis*, nasal polyps (fleshy growths that arise from the lining of the nasal and sinus passages), and an allergy to aspirin. These aspirin sensitive asthmatics are often the most difficult to treat.

The treatment of asthma combines the use of two types of medication: bronchodilators, usually in spray form, which open the narrowed bronchial tubes, plus anti-inflammatory agents that reduce irritation and swelling within the passageways. Several anti-inflammatory medications are available for the treatment of asthma but derivatives of the body hormone, cortisone, called corticosteroids or steroids, are the most potent anti-inflammatory agents available.

Bronchodilators are fast acting drugs that should be used only on an "as needed" basis. The ideal result of a successful asthma treatment regimen is when this type of medication is ultimately not needed at all. In contrast, the anti-inflammatory medication must be taken on a regular basis and often requires several days to achieve its effect. The need to use it regularly combined with the slower onset of action sometimes deters patients from using this form of medication. Too often patients become dependent on the rapidly acting bronchodilator sprays that provide nearly instant but only temporary relief for shortness of breath. When overused, the benefits of the bronchodilator diminish, so that an out-of-control asthmatic will typically spray more and more, to less and less benefit.

The most severely affected asthmatics who suffer frequent attacks often require high doses of corticosteroids given by mouth—or by injection if the patient is hospitalized. These medications have saved thousands of lives but this treatment, if given for a prolonged period, may have serious side effects including osteoporosis and the development of ulcerations in the digestive tract. Besides these and a long list of other adverse effects, the use of corticosteroids for prolonged periods often causes weight gain and the development of diabetes. Some patients develop a condition known as adrenal insufficiency in which the body's own source of cortisone, the adrenal glands, stop producing the hormone so that the patient becomes dependent on an external source. If medication is not administered to these patients, they may go into a state of near shock in which the blood pressure drops and vital organs shut down.

At about the time that I became a fellow in pulmonary diseases at Bellevue Hospital in 1973 a corticosteroid spray was introduced in this country. This break-through treatment allowed many patients who had been dependent on oral corticosteroids to use an inhaled form, which delivered the bulk of the medication to the bronchial tubes without being absorbed in large amounts into the whole body. Several additional inhaled corticosteroids quickly became available after 1973, some more potent than others; all provided the steroid benefit to the airways of asthmatics with much fewer adverse effects than oral corticosteroids.

Before our first visit Edith had received several courses of oral corticosteroids prescribed by her prior physicians for severe asthmatic attacks.

On our initial visit, she said, "I'll do anything you say, but don't give me steroids."

She was frightened by the side effects, having gained 10 pounds in the last year, which she attributed to the oral steroids. She was also concerned about other side effects.

"My mother had osteoporosis and she lost four inches in height. I don't want that to happen to me."

I promised to prescribe the oral form of this medication only if it was absolutely necessary and recommended the inhaled preparations. After listening to my explanation, she argued with me.

"They're still steroids, and you're telling me if I take them for a long time I may still get osteoporosis, is that right?"

I admitted there was a risk but it was only a low risk, and explained that by taking calcium and vitamin D supplements, this could be prevented. I cautioned that other potential side effects included a greater risk of cataracts and glaucoma had been found in elderly patients who used inhaled steroids.

"It sounds like these sprays aren't much better than the pills but I'll try them if you say so."

During our first visit I performed pulmonary function tests and found that Edith's bronchial tubes were severely constricted but showed improvement after she inhaled a bronchodilator. Her oxygen level was near normal as was her chest x-ray and routine laboratory tests.

I then told her my plan.

"I want to put together a regimen of medication for you to follow. The hardest thing for you will be to take medication when you feel well, but you must do it if you are to control your asthma."

I prescribed a bronchodilator spray, a non-steroidal anti-inflammatory agent known as cromolyn, which is taken by inhalation, plus an inhaled corticosteroid. Her medication list consisted of three different drugs.

"I know you think this is a lot of medication, but each drug has a specific role in keeping you well. I want you to return in one month so I can see how the medications are working. Also, please call me next week and give me a progress report."

Edith's first follow-up appointment was typical of many future visits.

"Dear doctor, how are you?"

Before I could inquire as to her progress, she went traveling on with her own train of thought.

"I've brought a copy of my latest journal for you to read."

Before I could respond, she would continue with such questions as, "What do you think of the situation in the Middle East?"

Suspecting that this was her way of avoiding coming to grips with what was required to deal with her chronic illness, I would then spend the next several minutes attempting to answer her question but eventually return to inquiries about her health. Many of these she deflected, but through my persistent questioning, I would finally learn that she had not been doing well.

On this particular visit she finally admitted that in the last month she had had to use her emergency bronchodilator spray several times a day. She also awakened several times during the nights with shortness of breath and wheezing. These signs were clear indications that her asthma was still out of control. I reexamined her lungs and heard wheezing so then repeated her pulmonary function tests. The results showed that her airways were still narrowed despite the treatment regimen I had put together.

Edith and I sat down together in my consultation room.

"It's clear from your symptoms, the exam, and breathing tests that you are not improving on these medications. It's going to be necessary to give you a short course of the oral corticosteroids to remove a lot of the inflammation in your airways. Once this is accomplished, we have a better chance of maintaining control over your asthma."

Her expression was one of disappointment and resistance.

"I don't want to take steroids."

I went over some of the potential consequences, including hospitalization and even the possibility of a fatal attack if she avoided the prescribed treatment.

"Very few people die of asthma but it can happen. You have a severe form of this disease which puts you at greater risk for serious asthmatic attacks, potentially fatal."

Edith thought for a while and finally tried to second-guess me.

"I don't think I'm really that ill but I have to trust your judgment. Can it be a very short course?"

"Edith, too little steroid will have much less effect and will last for a much shorter period of time. Please try doing it my way."

She finally agreed to follow my suggested 16-day steroid course. During this period she was to take the steroid medication only with or after food to minimize the chance of stomach irritation. I also asked her to avoid sweets and to increase the amount of potassium in her diet to prevent elevation of her blood sugar and muscle cramping that can be produced by corticosteroids.

On the next visit after her steroid course had ended Edith reported feeling much better, now sleeping through the night without asthmatic attacks and using her bronchodilator spray only about twice a week.

"The steroids worked," she announced, and then without missing a beat, "What do you think of the latest shenanigans of the CIA?"

Edith's politics and mine differed considerably with her being left of center and I being slightly to the right so some of our discussions were pretty lively.

One visit, while examining her lungs and reviewing her medications, I confided that I'd been a history major at Georgetown University and at one point considered a career in the Foreign Service instead of in medi-cine.

"Dear doctor, you would have been a wonderful diplomat! Look at how you convinced me to take those terrible steroids!" she chirped with enthu-siasm.

The course of Edith's asthma proved far from stable. Within three months she was back to using her bronchodilator spray too frequently and awakening at night. I added another asthma drug called theophylline to her treatment regimen and ordered a home nebulizer. A nebulizer is a sim-ple device that forces compressed air through liquid solutions of medica-tion producing a medicated mist or aerosol for inhalation. This device produces more inhaled medication than can be delivered by conventional asthma spray. Even with the addition of these medications, however, Edith's asthma remained out of control so I had to prescribe courses of oral steroids several times over the next few years.

With each course, Edith complained of weight gain and a change in the shape of her face characteristic of corticosteroid use, commonly known as a "moon face." She hated it.

"I must get off steroids. I am determined. Just look at my face and stomach."

I asked if she was using her steroid sprays regularly.

"Sometimes I skip them when I feel better," she answered reluctantly.

I pressed for more information. She parried with a commentary on cur-rent Eastern European politics, but finally revealed she had cut the dosage of the steroid sprays in half.

"Maybe one puff will work as well as two," she insisted.

I continued my mantra about the need to remain on regular medication to control her asthma.

"Edith, the benefits of inhaled steroids certainly outweighs the adverse effects. If you can maintain the inhaled steroids on a regular basis at the dosage I have prescribed, I don't think you'll need the oral steroids as much."

She seemed unconvinced, but gave in. "Dear doctor, I will do as you say."

I instructed her to increase the amount of the inhaled steroids and within two weeks she called to report that it was working, her attacks had diminished.

Soon after achieving better control over her asthma, Edith returned to ask me to reduce her medication.

"I don't want to be dependent on medication. Can't you take me off some of them? I'm thinking of trying some alternative treatments like Chinese herbs and acupuncture. What do you think?"

I explained that to reduce her medication might remove the control we had worked so long to achieve and that her asthmatic attacks would probably recur. She quickly changed the subject.

"Don't you think we should be doing more about human rights in communist China?"

I answered her original question instead.

"I have no problem with your trying acupuncture but I would stay away from any herbal remedies since we don't always know what's in them. I also recommend yoga because of the use of abdominal breathing and relaxation techniques. Why don't you try both of these alternative approaches and return in a few weeks. If your breathing tests improve, I will try to reduce your medication gradually."

I also asked her to consider working with a psychologist.

"You seem to have trouble accepting that you have a serious illness and it might help to talk to someone about this."

Edith seemed surprised at my suggestion.

"But dear doctor, there is nothing wrong with my mind. I just don't think that I'm as sick as you say. I can always find a way to control it."

I reminded her that she first saw me after an attack that had required emergency room treatment.

"Oh that was a mistake. I should never have been taken there. The attack really wasn't that bad."

A little over a month passed before she phoned again.

"I'm doing yoga and acupuncture and I have felt so much better lately that I stopped all of your medications a few days ago except for the bronchodilator spray and I still feel fine. I don't think I need them."

I was concerned that Edith had stopped her medications on her own and reminded her that we had planned a return office visit and a breathing test before her regimen was adjusted. Again, she didn't want my advice, just my reassurance that she was doing the right thing.

"I feel so well and it has been two days off those terrible drugs and I'm not wheezing at all."

I told her that some of her medications should have lingering effects for several days before they left her system completely and were probably still protecting her. She didn't want to hear that either.

"Did you see what's happening in North Korea? Isn't it awful?"

Frustrated, I finally asked her to call me back in another 48 hours to tell me how she was doing. She agreed.

It was less than 24 hours after this conversation that I received a call around midnight from the medical center's emergency room. Her neighbors had brought Edith to the ER with a severe asthmatic attack. I went to see her immediately and found her receiving oxygen and a nebulizer treatment. Her lung exam revealed severe wheezing.

"Dear Doctor, I am so sorry to get you out of bed. My friends overreacted; I could have just used my spray and stayed home. I hate causing you trouble."

I brushed her protestations aside and told her that her lung exam was much worse than usual and that she needed to stay in the hospital.

"Your oxygen level is lower than normal and you're wheezing. We have no choice but to put you back on corticosteroids, which will work faster if we give them intravenously. It was good that your neighbors brought you to the ER because when your oxygen level drops it means that this is a serious asthmatic attack."

Edith's expression was one of chagrin, disappointment and anxiety. At that moment one of the other patients in the ER suffered a cardiac arrest and a team of doctors began CPR. Edith was watching. Perhaps seeing what was going on gave my words more impact. She finally capitulated.

"I'll do as you say but please try to keep the steroids to a minimum."

We talked further about the risks of stopping medication on her own and she said, "I know it was wrong, but I hate taking medication, especially steroids, in any form."

How well I knew that. She didn't have to tell me!

Edith responded slowly to the intravenous steroids and the resumption of her medication routine. I saw her each day on rounds and her wheezing was gradually disappearing. After a week her chest sounded clear and she was ready for discharge so I went over her treatment regimen.

"You will be on the oral corticosteroids for two more weeks and you must continue your routine with the inhaled steroid sprays and other medications. This hospital junket can happen again if you cut down too fast or don't stick with the medication schedule."

"Oh no! I don't want to come back to the hospital, that's for sure. I am so unhappy when I'm not in my apartment. I miss my books."

On a follow-up appointment some time after her hospitalization I discovered another reason Edith was not taking her medications when she said, "These sprays are so expensive, I really can't afford them."

Although she edited the foreign policy journal, Edith was paid very little and lived mainly on social security. Her health insurance consisted of only Medicare and she was forced to pay the total cost of her medications out of her tiny monthly income.

It is not unusual for me to find that problem. Many of my Medicare patients describe the terrible choice that they must often make between eating and filling their prescriptions. At any given time a good number of my patients depend on samples I provide to maintain their medication routine.

"Edith, I receive samples of your medications from the pharmaceutical companies and I will try to keep you supplied as much as possible."

I literally had to coax Edith into taking the sample medications.

"Look, if you don't take them, they'll sit on the shelf and expire. You might as well take advantage of what I am given or else they'll go to waste."

Finally, she gave in.

For the next year, I kept Edith supplied with medication but she continued to cut back on their use whenever she felt better.

"I don't need so many drugs," she would say emphatically.

I would often hear the wheeze on examining her lungs during office visits and reminded her each time that she needed to be more regular with her medications. With each reminder she deflected my suggestions.

"I think I can control my asthma with my bronchodilator spray. It works much faster than anything else and it's not a steroid. You know, Dear Doctor, I am not afraid of dying, I had to face that every day when I was in the camps."

It was the first time in all our talks that Edith mentioned the concentration camp or death. I paused for a moment and said, "You survived that horror but why risk death now?"

"Oh Dear Doctor, you are always so concerned. I'll be fine. Let's not talk of death. Did you see my latest article?"

After Edith left I wondered that night if I'd stumbled onto the reason this highly intelligent woman repeatedly minimized her illness. Did asthma seem trivial in comparison to the Nazis and the death camps? Had her ability to survive the holocaust made her falsely confident that she could survive anything? Or was it that she carried guilt for surviving when so many others had not? Could it be that her deep down philosophy was stoicism—if her fate was to die from asthma, so be it? Had the loss of her husband brought on a depression, contributing to the ongoing denial of her illness?

I was never to learn the answer to these questions.

On a winter evening a few months later I received a call from a New York City policeman assigned to a Manhattan precinct.

"Doctor, I'm in the apartment of one of your patients, Edith Tannenbaum. I'm sorry to have to tell you—she's just died."

I asked him to tell me what had happened.

"According to her neighbors she entered the lobby of her apartment house around noon today, very short of breath and stopped to use her asthma spray. The doorman said he'd seen her in the same condition many times. He said that she would often come home wheezing, barely able to speak. After entering the lobby today he saw her take two puffs of her spray. A few minutes later she assured him, 'It's nothing to worry about; I just had to use my spray. The cold weather always makes me wheeze."

The policeman continued: "A few neighbors noticed that she was in distress as she entered her apartment. About an hour later one of those neighbors knocked on her door to see if she was okay, but there was no answer. Then we were called and we got here a few minutes later. I rapped at her door and there was no answer, so the building superintendent let us in."

The image of what he then described to me is with me still. After entering her apartment, the patrolman found Edith sitting in a chair very close to the door, still wearing her coat and hat. Clutched in her hand was her bronchodilator spray. It had to be pried loose by the medical examiner.

Reflecting to myself as I replaced the phone receiver, I spoke aloud. "Oh dear Edith, you could have survived this too."

EPILOGUE

From the beginnings of medicine, doctors have combined scientific knowledge with the art of healing. With the greater understanding of the functions of the human body and astounding breakthroughs like the decoding of the human genome, emphasis has been increasingly placed on technology and science. Objectivity has been applauded while empathy has been discouraged. This book has tried to demonstrate that diagnosis is both scientific and intuitive and that empathy may provide insight that improves treatment and the outcome of an illness.

The cases portrayed in this book are unusual but not unique. In each case, however, the doctor-patient relationship played a vital role. Kevin O'Connor outlived his predicted life expectancy many times over due to a strong bond that developed between himself and his physicians. Seth Howard used a survival mechanism from his childhood experience with polio and trusted his doctor's treatment plan because it "made sense." Mary Kelly faced a life-threatening illness at age 22 with the information from her physician that she needed to make her final days fulfilling. Katherine Cole's diagnosis of a rare fungal infection required a close bond between her and her physicians who were taught an important lesson. Recognition of Joseph Marino's "take charge" personality contributed to the quick discovery and treatment of his heart defect. Louis Goodman accepted treatment of his sleep apnea after intervention by another veteran brought to him by his physician. Despite the good outcomes of these cases, this book is also meant to illustrate that every physician knows failure and disappointment. Edith Tannenbaum continued to deny her illness and died of a treatable disease just after revealing a clue to the source of her denial.

In all of these seven cases, empathy provided added insight and knowledge. This is much more than sympathy for another individual's pain or suffering. In medicine empathy starts with interest on the part of the physician who takes a detailed history from his patient. The physician must be able to listen carefully and to communicate openly. He must also be a keen observer of his patient's moods and reactions. The histories include life experiences as well as the description of the illness at hand. They are often moving, producing a strong emotional response. Visual images are generated and the observer begins to instantly recognize his subject's mood changes. The emotions generated promote increased self-awareness and discovery on the part of the physician.

Can empathy be learned? I feel that my own experience is proof that it can. Although my education started early by observing my father's close interaction with his patients, I continued to learn from many other physician role models who practiced medicine by first listening and communicating. Medical schools now begin student-patient interaction much earlier in their curriculums. In an important exercise, students are often placed in the role of a patient to experience firsthand what this means.

Why are so many patients dissatisfied with their physicians? Surveys of patients reveal that it is often a failure on the part of the physician to communicate. It is common to find patients changing from one physician to the next, searching for "someone who cares" or "someone I can talk to" and especially "someone who will listen."

Communication takes time. It is not surprising to find that physicians are also dissatisfied. In the current era of managed care, they are often forced to see large numbers of patients in shortened visits in order to offset higher expenses and reduced fee schedules, leaving less and less time for patient-doctor interaction.

Can this trend be reversed? The answer is unclear. It will require physicians to manage their time better with innovative techniques such as voice recognition software to document their findings and support staff to perform certain tasks, i.e. recording vital signs, filling out forms, etc. The time gained from these steps can then be used for patient-doctor interaction. HMOs must also be made aware of the impact of their policies and fee schedules on patient care. They must be responsive to the value of the time a physician spends taking a detailed history, performing exams, teaching, and answering questions. Fee schedules that have heavily favored technical procedures must be revised and balanced to validate the time invested by the physician at the bedside. Our health care system is in turmoil but it can be repaired. It will require both doctors and patients to take their complaints to the HMOs and their elected representatives.

How should you choose a physician? A great deal of information on physician qualifications such as board certification and "Best Doctor" listings is now available and is included in the Appendix. The experiences of the patients recounted in this book provide practical advice. Seth Howard's history illustrates that trust in your physician is of the utmost importance. A lack of satisfaction may lead a patient to change physicians or seek a second opinion as Mary Kelly did. Kevin O'Connor's "never give up" attitude told him not to accept the opinion of two specialists and to seek a third opinion. Only by spending time with your physician can you assess whether there is good communication and rapport. If a physician is unable to provide this time or fails to meet your needs, then another choice must be made.

The cases recorded in this book demonstrate that medicine isn't entirely objective and scientific. The emotions physicians experience are natural and should not be suppressed since they may offer insight into patients' illnesses. Through this better understanding of his patient, empathy may empower a doctor to offer a more suitable treatment and help him to "heal." This may not be a cure but may simply be the achievement of comfort and peace.

GLOSSARY

Acidosis: Excess acid in the blood and body.

Air Sacs: Alveoli.

Allergen: Substance producing an allergic reaction.

Allergy: Hypersensitivity to a specific substance.

Alveoli: Tiny air sacs that make up lung tissue in which the exchange of oxygen and carbon dioxide occur.

Apnea: Temporary cessation of breathing of at least ten seconds.

ASD: Atrial septal defect. Opening between the two upper chambers of the heart.

Asthma: A disease of the air passages of the lung in which the bronchial tubes become inflamed and hyperirritable.

Atelectasis: Lung condition in which the air sacs, or alveoli, are collapsed preventing the exchange of oxygen and carbon dioxide with the blood.

Atria: The upper chambers of the heart.

Biopsy: Examination of tissue or cells removed from a living person for the purpose of diagnosis.

BIPAP: Bilevel positive airway pressure device providing positive pressure delivered by a face or nasal mask. This device assists in the work of breathing.

Blood Gas: Measures the levels of oxygen (O2) and carbon dioxide (CO2) from a sample of blood from an artery.

Bronchitis: Inflammation of the bronchial tubes.

Bronchoscopy: Procedure in which a lighted scope, called a bronchoscope, is introduced into the lungs through the bronchial tubes.

Bullae: Large cyst-like spaces between the lung's air sacs: from the Latin, a bubble.

Bullous: Type of emphysema in which large cysts (bullae) occur.

Carbon Dioxide (CO2): Waste product of body metabolism, gas excreted by the lungs in exhalation.

CAT Scan: Abbreviation for computerized axial tomography. Combination of x-ray and computer program produces a cross-sectional image.

Central Sleep Apnea: Sleep apnea caused by the respiratory center in the brain failing to trigger breathing.

Chemotherapy: Treatment of disease by means of chemicals or drugs.

Cilia: Rod-like extensions of the lining cells of the bronchial tubes. Sweeping motion of the cilia causes mucus to move upward toward the throat, from which it may be expectorated.

Clubbing: Condition affecting the fingers and toes characterized by increased curvature of the nails and widened and thickened digits.

CPAP: Abbreviation for continuous positive airway pressure. An air pressure device that uses the flow of air to maintain the opening of the throat.

Craniotomy: Procedure in which a piece of the skull is removed permitting wider exposure of the brain.

Cryptococcosis: Infection with a fungus or yeast known as cryptococcosis neoformans.

Cyanosis: Dark blue or purplish discoloration of the skin, nail beds, and lips due to a deficiency of oxygen in the blood.

DNA: Abbreviation for deoxyribonucleic acid, the compound that contains the genetic code of living tissue.

Dyspnea: Air hunger resulting in labored or difficult breathing: from the Greek meaning bad breathing.

Echocardiogram (Echo): Non-invasive diagnostic procedure that uses ultrasound to visualize cardiac structures.

Edema: Excess fluid in the tissues.

Edematous: Swelling; affected with edema.

Elastase: An enzyme that breaks down elastin, a protein found in tissue, destroying the walls of the air sacs, resulting in emphysema.

Electrocardiogram (EKG): Record of the electrical activity of the heart.

Emphysema: Lung disease in which walls of air sacs are destroyed and supporting structure of bronchial tubes is weakened.

Erythropoetin: A hormone that stimulates red blood cell production.

Expiration: Relating to breathing out or exhaling.

Hemoglobin: Protein substance contained in the red blood cell that transports oxygen to the tissues.

Hemoptysis: Blood-spitting.

Hypertrophic Osteoarthopathy: Presence of bulbous deformity of the tip of the fingers generally known as digital clubbing.

Inspiration: Inhalation of air.

Iron Lung: Metal tank or cylinder designed to assist breathing by producing a vacuum or negative pressure around the outside of the chest, mimicking normal action of breathing.

Lobes: Divisions of the lungs.

Lymph Glands: Part of the body's immune system.

Meningiomas: Benign growths arising from the outer covering of the brain.

Meningitis: Infection of the membranes (meninges) that cover the brain and spinal cord.

Metabolism: The sum of the chemical changes of the body in which nutrients are broken down and used for body functions.

Metastases: Movement of body cells, especially cancer cells, from one part of the body to another.

MRI: Clear images of the body through the use of a large magnet, radio waves, and a computer.

Mucosa: Mucous membrane covering inner surface of many structures of the body, including the nose and bronchial tubes.

Myocardial Infarction: Heart attack.

Neurons: Nerve cells.

Neutrophils: Type of white blood cell often involved in immune reactions.

Obstructive: A form of sleep apnea due to a closure of the muscles that support the throat.

Oncologist: Cancer specialist.

Oximeter: Device measuring saturation or enrichment of the blood with oxygen.

OSA: Obstructive sleep apnea.

Oxygen (O2): Gas needed for life-sustaining activities of the body; taken up by red blood cells in the walls of the alveoli.

Phlegm: Mucus.

Pneumonectomy: Surgical removal of an entire lung.

Poliomyelitis: Viral infection that attacks the nervous system, disabling muscles and sometimes suffocating its victims.

Polysomnography: Non-invasive monitoring of sleep.

Positive Pressure Respirator: Delivery of forced air to the lungs by a mechanical ventilator.

PPS: Post polio syndrome seen in survivors of paralytic polio. PPS symptoms are usually weakness, fatigue, and pain.

Pulmonary Angiogram: Procedure to detect pulmonary embolism by a radiographic examination of the pulmonary circulation following injection of a contrast agent.

Pulmonary Embolus: Blood clot that travels through the circulation to lodge in a blood vessel in the lung.

Pulmonary Function Tests: Measurements taken to determine lung capacity and performance.

Pulmonologist: Internist with specialized training in lung disease.

Radiation Therapy: Delivery of intense heat directed at a specific site of malignancy.

Radon: Second leading cause of lung cancer. A radioactive gas that forms when uranium naturally breaks down in rock, soil or water.

REM: Rapid eye movement. Cyclic movement of the closed eyes observed during sleep. Accounts for 25 percent of sleep time.

Respirator: From the Latin to breathe. A mechanical method of assisting breathing.

Rhinitis: Inflammation of nasal membranes or lining. Rhinitis may be allergic or non-allergic.

Sarcoma: Malignant tumor. A rare cancer that arises from soft tissue of the body.

Scoliosis: Curvature of the spine producing a restriction in the expansion of the lungs.

Sciatica: Pain from pressure on the sciatic nerve.

Shunt: To divert.

Sleep Apnea: Periodic cessation of breathing during sleep.

Spinal Tap (lumbar puncture): Procedure to sample spinal fluid to confirm meningitis.

TEE: Transesophageal echocardiography. Obtains a more detailed image of the heart by placing an electrode in the esophagus.

Thoracoscopic Surgery: Video guided surgery of the chest similar to a laparoscopic operation on the abdomen.

Thoracotomy: Surgical incision of the chest wall.

Trachea: Main air passage, or windpipe, beginning below the voice box (larynx); divides into right and left main bronchial tubes.

Tracheotomy: Opening through the neck and into the trachea, through which a tube is inserted to create an airway.

Uvula: Soft cone-like projection from the soft palate.

Ventricles: Lower chambers of the heart.

Vital Capacity: Total amount of air in the lungs after maximum inhalation.

APPENDIX

RESOURCES ON THE INTERNET

FINDING A DOCTOR

American Medical Association
 www.ama-assn.org
Doctor finder. A complete listing of doctors and their medical background.

Castle Connolly's America's Top Doctors
 www.castleconnolly.com
Search profiles of the best doctors and hospitals. There is no charge for a limited search but a full search requires a payment of $21.95, which covers one year.

Medicare—U.S. Government Site for People with Medicare
 www.medicare.gov
A listing of physicians participating in Medicare. Participating physicians accept assignment.

FINDING HEALTH INFORMATION

Healthfinder
 www.healthfinder.gov
Guide to reliable health information; available in Spanish.

Internet Drug Index
www.rxlist.com
Provides information on medications including adverse effects. This site includes a health library for specific diseases and lists the drugs that are indicated for treatment.

MedlinePlus—Service of the U.S. National Library and National Institutes of Health
www.medlineplus.gov
This site lists health topics, drug information, medical encyclopedia and dictionary and includes directories to help you find a doctor, dentist and hospital.

WebMDHealth
www.mywebmd.com
This site has a medical library with information on health topics including explanations of diagnostic tests.

RESOURCES—BOOKS

All I Want Is A Good Night's Sleep
Author: Sonia Ancoli-Israel. PhD
Publisher: Mosby; lst edition
  Strategies for dealing with sleep disorders.

The Asthma Sourcebook
Author: Francis V. Adams, MD
Publisher: McGraw-Hill/Contemporary Books; 2nd edition
  Everything you need to know about asthma.

The Breathing Disorders Sourcebook
Author: Francis V. Adams, MD
Publisher: McGraw-Hill/Contemporary Books
  Everything you need to know about breathing and its disorders.

Cancer: 50 Essential Things To Do
Author: Greg Anderson, O. Carl Simonton, MD
Publisher: Plume; Revised and updated edition
  Useful information from a cancer survivor.

Coping With Prednisone
Author: Eugenia Zukerman, Julie Ingelfinger, MD
Publisher: Griffin Trade Paperback
  How to handle the side effects of cortisone.

Health Smart: Hospital Handbook
Author: Joseph Sacco, MD
Publisher: Alpha Books
  How to survive a hospital stay.

Medical Language Instant Translator
Author: Davi-Ellen Chabner
Publisher: W. B. Saunders
  Translates medical terms into everyday English.

Merck Manual of Medical Information
Author: Mark H. Beers, MD; Editor in Chief
Publisher: Simon & Schuster; 2nd edition
  Comprehensive medical reference book.

Patients Guide to Medical Tests
Author: Joseph Segen, MD; Joseph Stauffer, PhD
Publisher: Checkmark Books; 2nd edition
  Explanations of common medical tests.

RESOURCES—ORGANIZATIONS

American Lung Association
61 Broadway, 6th Floor
New York, NY 10006
(212) 315-8700
www.lungusa.org
A highly informative national organization with local chapters throughout the United States. You can locate your local chapter by calling 1-800-LUNG-USA.

American Sleep Apnea Association
1424 K Street NW, Suite 302
Washington, DC 20005
(202) 293-3650
www.sleepapnea.org
An organization dedicated to enhancing the well-being of those affected by sleep apnea.

Joint Commission on Accreditation of Healthcare Organizations (JCAHO)
One Renaissance Blvd.
Oakbrook Terrace, IL 60181
(630) 792-5000
www.jcaho.org
You may report a concern or complaint about the quality of care at a health care organization and check to see if they are accredited.

National Institutes of Health (NIH)
9000 Rockville Pike
Betheseda, MD 20894
(301) 496-4000
  www.nih.gov
U.S. government's major center for health research. This web site links to
its twenty-seven institutes and centers.

National Jewish Medical and Research Center
1400 Jackson Street
Denver, CO 80206
1-800-222-LUNG
  www.njc.org
World-renowned medical center for research, evaluation and treatment of
pulmonary diseases.

Post-Polio Health International
4201 Lindell Boulevard #110
Saint Louis, Missouri 63108-2915
(314) 534-0475
  www.post-polio.org
Organization with the goal of enhancing the lives of polio survivors
through education, advocacy and research.

U.S. Environmental Protection Agency (EPA)
Ariel Rios Building
1200 Pennsylvania Avenue, N.W.
Washington, DC 20460
(202) 272-0167
  www.epa.gov
Indoor air quality information including radon, the second leading cause
of lung cancer.

U.S. Food and Drug Administration (FDA)
5600 Fishers Lane
Rockville, MD 20857-0001
(310) 827-6250; (888)-463-6332
 www.fda.gov
Information on drugs, food, medical devices, market recalls and safety alerts.

0-595-31626-3

www.ingramcontent.com/pod-product-compliance
Lightning Source LLC
Chambersburg PA
CBHW020256290526
45784CB00003B/1272